Anticoagulation - Current Perspectives

Edited by Xingshun Qi and Xiaozhong Guo

Published in London, United Kingdom

Anticoagulation - Current Perspectives
http://dx.doi.org/10.5772/intechopen.98119
Edited by Xingshun Qi and Xiaozhong Guo

Contributors
Ibrahim Kalle Kwaifa, José López-Castro, Isabel Izuzquiza Avanzini, Raquel Gutiérrez-López, Manuel Lorenzo López Reboiro, Clara Martínez Vivero, Iris Bararu Bojan, Stefan Dobreanu, Oana-Viola Badulescu, Maria Cristina Vladeanu, Andrei Bojan, Carmen Elena Plesoianu, Manuela Ciocoiu, Ortigoza Daniel Victor, Ana Paula Callejo de Souza, Franciele Cordeiro Gabriel, Géssica Caroline Henrique Fontes-Mota, Mariana de Siqueira Siva, Eliane Ribeiro, Harry N. Magnani

First published in London, United Kingdom, 2022 by IntechOpen
IntechOpen is the global imprint of INTECHOPEN LIMITED, registered in England and Wales, registration number: 11086078, 5 Princes Gate Court, London, SW7 2QJ, United Kingdom

British Library Cataloguing-in-Publication Data
A catalogue record for this book is available from the British Library

Additional hard and PDF copies can be obtained from orders@intechopen.com

Anticoagulation - Current Perspectives
Edited by Xingshun Qi and Xiaozhong Guo
p. cm.
Print ISBN 978-1-80355-891-2
Online ISBN 978-1-80355-892-9
eBook (PDF) ISBN 978-1-80355-893-6

For EU product safety concerns:
IN TECH d.o.o., Prolaz Marije Krucifikse Kozulić 3, 51000 Rijeka, Croatia,
info@intechopen.com or visit our website at intechopen.com.

Meet the editors

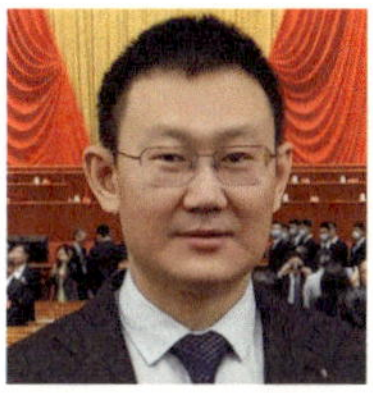

Dr. Xingshun Qi is a deputy director at the Department of Gastroenterology, General Hospital of Northern Theater Command, China (formerly General Hospital of Shenyang Military Area). His major research interests are the management of liver cirrhosis, portal hypertension (especially portal vein thrombosis and Budd-Chiari syndrome), and hepatocellular carcinoma. He has edited eight English-language books and serves as an associate editor for *BMC Gastroenterology*, an associate editor for *Frontiers in Medicine*, an academic editor for *Canadian Journal of Gastroenterology and Hepatology*, an editorial board member of *Therapeutic Advances in Gastroenterology*, and an advisory editorial member of *Advances in Therapy*.

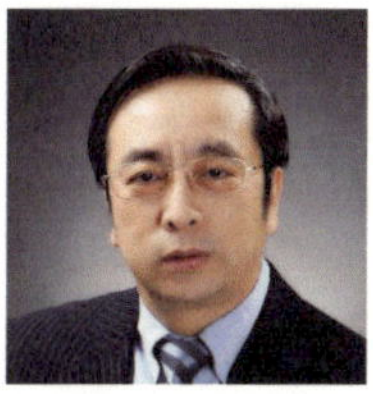

Prof. Xiaozhong Guo is the director of the Department of Gastroenterology, General Hospital of Northern Theater Command, China(formerly General Hospital of Shenyang Military Area). He has practiced in the field of digestive diseases and digestive endoscopy for more than thirty years. His major achievements include experimental and clinical research on the management of pancreatic diseases, especially pancreatic cancer, and stem cells for digestive diseases such as liver cirrhosis and ulcerative colitis. He has published more than 500 papers and edited more than ten books. He has received six funds from the National Natural Science Foundation of China. He received first prizes from the *Natural Science* and *Science and Technology Progress Awards* of Liaoning Province.

Contents

Preface

Nowadays, thrombotic diseases are some of the leading causes of death in the world. Anticoagulation is a mainstay approach for the prophylaxis and treatment of thrombotic diseases. The clinical requirement of drugs with greater efficacy and lower risk of bleeding complications has prompted investigators to conduct experimental and clinical research on the development and validation of new anticoagulants. To date, there are three major types of commonly used anticoagulants. The first type is vitamin K antagonists (VKAs), including warfarin and acenocoumarol; the second type is heparins, including unfractionated heparin, low molecular weight heparin, such as dalteparin and enoxaparin, and fondaparinux sodium; and the third type is direct oral anticoagulants (DOACs), including apixaban, dabigatran, edoxaban, and rivaroxaban. Knowledge regarding the use of anticoagulants has rapidly expanded in recent years. Accordingly, it is important to collect available evidence and summarize the current perspectives on anticoagulation. This book, *Anticoagulation - Current Perspectives*, includes six chapters regarding the mechanisms of anticoagulation and its clinical value in different disease conditions. The first two chapters summarize the general information regarding anticoagulation and hypercoagulability/thrombophilia, and the remaining four chapters discuss the use of anticoagulation in different populations, including adult hospitalized surgical and medical patients, COVID-19 patients, patients with hepatic thrombotic disorders, and frail elderly patients with atrial fibrillation. I hope that this book will be helpful for physicians to more deeply understand when and how patients should undergo anticoagulation and to further improve patient outcomes.

Dr. Xingshun Qi
Department of Gastroenterology,
General Hospital of Northern Theater Command,
Shenyang, China

Xiaozhong Guo
Professor,
Department of Gastroenterology,
General Hospital of Northern Theater Command,
Shenyang, China

Section 1

General Summary

Chapter 1

Anticoagulants and Hypercoagulability

Ibrahim Kalle Kwaifa

Abstract

Anticoagulants are chemical substances that prevent coagulation or prolong the clotting time by suppressing the functions or synthesis of coagulation factors in the blood. Anticoagulation mechanisms are essential in controlling the formation of a blood clot at the site of injury. The abnormalities in the coagulation and fibrinolytic mechanisms could lead to a hypercoagulability state. Inherited hypercoagulable state due, including Factor V Leiden (FVL), prothrombin gene mutation, defective natural proteins that inhibit coagulation, including antithrombin III (ATIII), protein C and S, high levels of FVII, FIX and FXI, are well-documented. Abnormalities of the fibrinolytic system, including tissue-type plasminogen activator (t-PA) and urokinase plasminogen activator (u-PA), and elevated levels of plasminogen activator inhibitor-1 (PAI-1) have been linked to hypercoagulation. Acquired conditions, including certain cancers and their medications, trauma or surgery, pregnancy, obesity and hyperlipidaemia, have been implicated with hypercoagulable events. The clinical symptoms of hypercoagulability can be devastating and may even have lethal outcomes. This activity reviews the principles of anticoagulation, haemostasis, deficiencies associated with hypercoagulability (both coagulation and fibrinolytic disorders), mechanisms of action of some natural-based products with anticoagulant potentials and highlights new clinical and traditional therapeutic strategies to be taken in improving healthcare for patients demanding anticoagulation.

Keywords: anticoagulants, coagulation and fibrinolytic system, hypercoagulability

1. Introduction

Haemostasis is a protective process that regulates and maintains stable physiology in the system. The physiology of haemostasis is extremely complex and reflects a delicate balance between the constant blood flow and immediate localised response to vascular injury. The process of haemostasis is traditionally divided into a cellular phase (involving platelets), known as the primary haemostatic phase and a fluid phase (involving plasma proteins), also called the secondary haemostatic phase [1]. It associates with other body defence mechanisms, including the immune system and the inflammatory responses [2]. During vascular injury, the increased blood pressure exerted in the blood circulation requires powerful and regulated localised pro-coagulant responses to minimise blood loss without compromising blood flow. Systemic anticoagulant and fibrinolytic components in other ways are also developed to inhibit the extension of the pro-coagulant responses to escalate beyond the vascular endothelial control, which may result in thrombotic formation. Thus, the haemostatic system is defined as a complex, highly regulated and integrated process, comprising both activators and inhibitory pathways, including blood vessels, platelets activities, coagulation and fibrinolytic system together [3]. While the coagulation cascade is aimed at fibrin formation through the production of thrombin, which is converted to fibrinogen (FN) and subsequently to fibrin, in the fibrinolytic system, plasmin is the main enzyme that plays a key role in dissolving the already formed clots by degrading fibrin. Physiological anticoagulation mechanisms function to suppress thrombin generation or inhibit its effects. Alterations to these mechanisms could lead to hypercoagulable states. This chapter will focus on the mechanisms associated with anticoagulation and defects of the anticoagulation mechanisms, leading to hypercoagulable states. The review also gave a concise description of the clinical approaches and traditional intervention to minimise the effects of hypercoagulability, which may progress to cardiovascular diseases (CVDs).

2. Haemostasis

2.1 The crosstalk between coagulation cascade and fibrinolytic system

Knowledge of the universal sequence of events in haemostasis can give vital information to the progress and development of thrombosis [4]. Within the blood coagulation cascade, the extrinsic pathway is mostly activated by vascular endothelial injury. In contrast, the intrinsic pathway is triggered solely through Factor XII (FXII) exposure on the thrombogenic surface. Even though separated, these pathways are interconnected at several points [4]. Both extrinsic and intrinsic pathways are linked to initiating the common pathway, which terminates at the formation of fibrin clots that are subsequently degraded by plasmin during fibrinolysis (**Figure 1**) [5]. Within the damaged endothelium, platelet adhesion and activation are promoted by the extremely exposed thrombogenic subendothelial extracellular matrix (ECM). Through its interactions with proconvertin (FVII), tissue factor (TF) initiates the coagulation cascade by converting prothrombin to thrombin. During secondary haemostasis, the thrombin generated triggers FN generation, which is converted to an insoluble fibrin plug that formed a fibrin mesh network together with aggregated platelets [4]. These assist to stop the blood flow, thus ensuring "haemostasis" and the final step of the coagulation cascade [6]. At the "thrombus", the circulating blood cells become trapped into the fibrin structure, and fibrin cross-linked is accomplished by Factor XIII activator (FXIIIa), which is promoted by the thrombin, leading to solid structural stability and the initial step of the fibrinolytic system [7].

During the repair process, the generated thrombus is destroyed by plasmin activities, produced by its zymogen plasminogen, tissue-type plasminogen activator (t-PA) or uPA on the fibrin clot [8]. Proteolysis of fibrin generates soluble fibrin degradation products (FDPs). The fibrinolytic system is extremely controlled by a protease enzyme inhibitor known as plasminogen activator inhibitor-1 (PAI-1), synthesised by endothelium, adipose tissue and the liver. The PAI-1 serves as a potent irreversible inhibitor of plasminogen activators, including t-PA and uPA, which convert plasminogen to plasmin, to promote fibrinolysis. The major plasminogen activator is t-PA, which has a high affinity to fibrin. The t-PA is secreted by endothelial cells or synthesised locally following the activation of endothelium by histamine, adrenalin, thrombin, FXa and hypoxia [9].

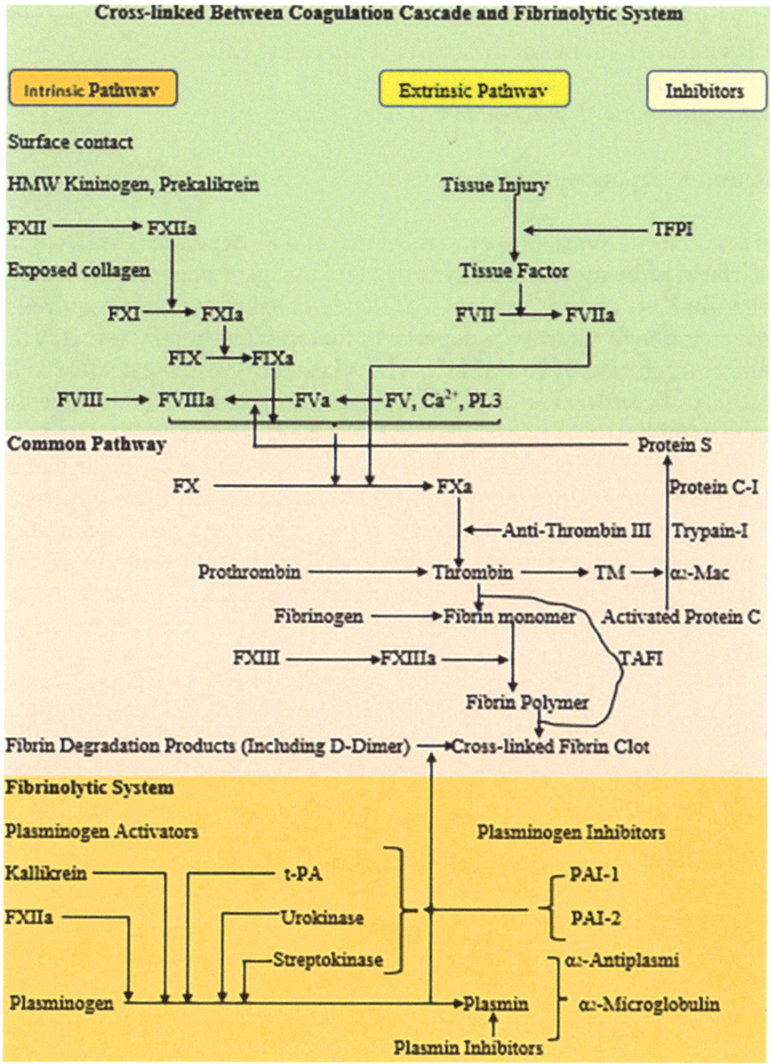

Figure 1.
Coagulation cascade and its interrelationship with the fibrinolytic system. Both extrinsic and intrinsic pathways of the coagulation cascade join to initiate the activation of FX of the common pathway. These unite to a fibrin clot, which is eventually degraded by plasmin in the fibrinolytic system.

The u-PA is another plasminogen activator secreted by several cells, such as fibroblasts, epithelial cells and the placenta. The indigenous form of uPA is transformed into a two-chain protein by plasmin or following stimulation by the contact factors, such as FXII, prekallikrein and high molecular weight kininogen (HMWK) (**Figure 1**) [10]. The uPA and t-PA convert plasminogen into plasmin through urokinase plasminogen activator-receptor (uPA-R) and LDL-receptor related protein-1 (LRP-1) respectively [11].

2.2 Anticoagulants and the mechanisms of action

Generally, anticoagulants exert their effects at different points of the coagulation cascade. Certain anticoagulants function directly as enzyme inhibitors, while some act indirectly by binding to antithrombin (AT) or inhibiting their production in the liver, such as vitamin K-dependent factors (**Figure 2**) [12].

2.2.1 The mode of actions of the common anticoagulants

I. Vitamin K dependent anticoagulant

Coumarin and its derivatives are a class of vitamin K–dependent anticoagulants (VKAs). Warfarin is the most common anticoagulant agent currently in use. It functions to inhibit vitamin K epoxide reductase (VKOR), which is necessarily required for the gamma-carboxylation of vitamin K-dependent factor, including factors II, VII, IX, X and protein C and S. Inhibition of vitamin K carboxylation triggers the decreased hepatic synthesis activity of clotting factors, leading to an anticoagulated state. Bleeding is the most common complication associated with warfarin therapy and is related to exponentially higher international normalised ratio (INR) values. The goal of the management is to reduce the INR back to a therapeutic safe level and hence are monitored by the value of the INR [13]. The dose-effect is narrow, and its actions are altered intensely by some factors, such as vegetables, greenleaf, some certain fruits, some drugs while inherited mutations in the VKOR complex may lead to resistance [12].

II. Unfractionated heparin (UFH)

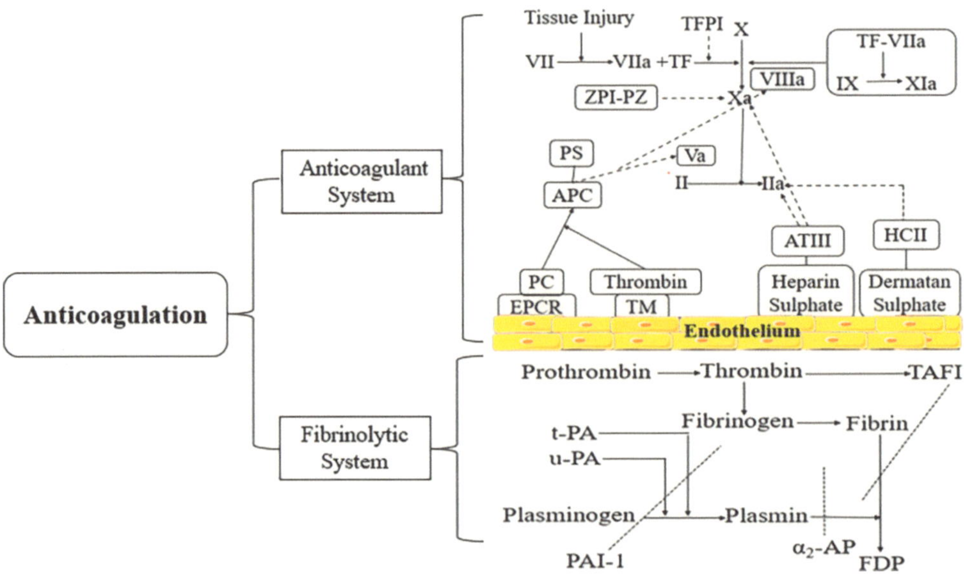

Figure 2.
Mechanisms of Anticoagulation. The anticoagulation system inhibits coagulation through a delicate balance between the activators and inhibitors of the coagulation cascade. At the fibrinolytic system, the balance between the activators of the fibrinolysis, including t-PA and u-PA and inhibitors, such as PAI-1 and α2-AP ensures the inhibition of fibrin formation or immediate dissolution of fibrin when it is formed. TF; tissue factor, TFPI; tissue factor pathway inhibitor, TAFI; thrombin activatable fibrinolysis inhibitor, EPCR; endothelial protein C receptor, ZPI; protein Z-dependent protease inhibitor, PZ; protein Z, TM; thrombomodulin, PC; protein C, APC; activated protein C, PS; protein S, HCII; heparin cofactor II, TM; thrombomodulin, t-PA; tissue-type plasminogen, u-PA; urokinase-type plasminogen activator, PAI-1; plasminogen activator inhibitor-1, α2-AP; α2-antiplasmin, FDP; fibrin degradation products. The dashed arrows indicate inhibition while thick arrow lines indicate activation.

Heparin forms a complex with antithrombin III (ATIII) and inactivates several coagulation factors, including FVII. It has a rapid onset of action and a short half-life. Heparin is monitored by activated partial thromboplastin time (aPTT) and anti-Factor Xa activity. The ratio of 1.5–2.2 times is the recommended target for aPTT [12].

III. Low molecular weight heparin (LMWH)

Nadroparin, enoxaparin, and tinzaparin have a shorter half-life compared to UFH. However, LMWH is not necessarily monitored unless in some conditions, such as pregnancy and renal failure [12].

IV. Fondaparinux sodium

Fondaparinux sodium also called "Arixtra", is a new class of synthetic pentasaccharide anticoagulants that bind to ATIII and indirectly inhibit the action of factor Xa. It has a similar mode of action to LMWH but has a longer half-life (17–21 h) than heparin. It does not prevent thrombin generation or interact with platelets but could be an essential and effective alternative to LMWH for the treatment of VTE following an orthopaedic surgical procedure. Fondaparinux is administered subcutaneously and excreted by unsaturated renal filtration [1].

V. Idrabiotaparinux sodium

Idrabiotaparinux sodium is another related family also injected subcutaneously once a week. It has a similar chemical structure and mode of action as fondaparinux but with a half-life of about 5–6 times longer than fondaparinux (fondaparinux's 17 hours to about 80 hours), indicating that the drug needs to be administered only once a week. The biotin attached to its structure allows its neutralisation with avidin, an egg-derived protein with low antigenicity [2].

VI. Inhibitors of FXa

Rivaroxaban, apixaban, edoxaban, betrixaban, apixaban and edoxaban are the common types of FXa inhibitors. They act by inhibiting the cleavage of prothrombin to thrombin through binding to FXa. They do not usually require constant monitoring [14].

VII. Inhibitors of thrombin

Bivalirudin and dabigatran are common examples of thrombin inhibitors. They act by inhibiting the cleavage of FN to fibrin and are metabolised in the kidney [12].

2.3 Important pathways associated with anticoagulation mechanisms

2.3.1 In the anticoagulant system

Protein C pathway: Protein C is a vitamin K-dependent serine protease produced in the liver and metabolised to its active form, known as activated protein C (APC) by thrombin. It is a strong anticoagulant that degrades FVa and FVIIIa and limits the coagulation process. The effect of APC is hindered by protein C inhibitors, such as α_2- macroglobulin and α_1-antitrypsin [15].

Thrombomodulin (TM) is a trans-membrane receptor available on endothelial cells. TM binds to thrombin to form a TM–thrombin complex that increases the synthesis of APC through which thrombin efficiently functions as an anticoagulant, that inhibits clot generation on the undamaged endothelium area [15].

Protein S is a vitamin K-dependent glycoprotein produced by hepatocytes and endothelial cells. It acts as cofactor to APC in the deactivation of FVa and FVIIIa. It is available in the plasma in many forms but only the free form shows anticoagulant activity. It also has anticoagulant activities independent of APC, such as direct reversible suppression of the prothrombinase (FVa–FXa) complex [15].

Tissue factor pathway inhibitor (TFPI) is a polypeptide synthesised by the endothelial cells and circulates in the plasma. It is the major inhibitor of the TF pathway, named the extrinsic pathway. It inhibits the coagulation cascade through the binding of the circulating FVIIa, that has been exposed to TF. It also binds to FXa to establish a TFPI–FXa complex, which reversibly inhibited FXa. Protein S facilitates the reaction between the TFPI and FXa in the presence of calcium ions and phospholipid, the activity of which is independent of APC [15].

Protein Z-dependent protease inhibitor (ZPI) has been recently identified as the component of the anticoagulant system. It is a plasma enzyme synthesised by the liver. It suppresses FXa activities in an interaction that involves both PZ and calcium. The PZ is a vitamin K-dependent glycoprotein and acts as a cofactor for ZPI [15].

2.3.2 In the fibrinolytic system

Plasmin or plasminogen is the major enzyme of the fibrinolytic system produced in the liver, as plasminogen proenzyme is released into the circulation. Although it could not cleave fibrin but has an affinity to fibrin, which is incorporated in the clot and transformed to plasmin through the t-PA and u-PA. Plasmin acts as a serine protease that cleaves fibrin to form soluble FDP. Plasmin exhibits positive feedback on its production [15].

Plasminogen activators: The t-PA is a serine protease that is released into the blood through the damaged endothelial cells. It binds to fibrin and converts clot-bound plasminogen to plasmin. The t-PA significantly contribute to the dissolution of fibrin and the maintenance of vascular integrity. The u-PA is found in the blood and ECM. It binds to a specific cell surface receptor known as the u-PAR, which stimulate the cell-bound plasminogen [15].

Fibrin as a cofactor: t-PA and plasminogen can bind to fibrin and form a tertiary complex, which is essential for plasmin formation. Thus, fibrin serves a dual purpose as a cofactor for plasminogen activation and a final substrate for plasmin generation. The partly degraded fibrin by plasmin offers much more efficient binding sites for plasminogen, which allows for the deposition of plasminogen on the clot, resulting in facilitated plasmin formation clot lysis [16].

Inhibitors of fibrinolysis (plasminogen activator inhibitors): The PAIs inhibit the progress of plasminogen to plasmin. Many types of PAIs have been identified and documented, but PAI type-1 has been investigated as the major physiological inhibitor. It is a glycoprotein produced by several cell types, such as megakaryocytes, endothelial cells, hepatocytes, and adipocytes. PAI-1 suppresses fibrinolysis by irreversibly inhibiting t-PA and u-PA. PAI-1 is taken up during the process and thus described as a 'suicide inhibitor' [16].

The a_2-Antiplasmin (a_2-AP) is the main inhibitor of plasmin. It is a circulating glycoprotein synthesis by the liver, which suppresses plasmin activity in one of the fastest proteins–protein interactions. The α_2-Macroglobulin is also produced by the liver and has been recognised as the secondary inhibitor of plasmin in plasma. It functions to deactivate plasminogen activators, APC, and thrombin [16].

Thrombin activatable fibrinolysis inhibitor (TAFI) is a plasma proenzyme that is produced by the liver and described as procarboxypeptidase U (unstable procarboxypeptidase), plasma procarboxypeptidase B, or procarboxypeptidase R. It is stimulated to carboxypeptidase by thrombin. TAFIa creates a useful link between coagulation and fibrinolytic systems. It removes lysine (and arginine) residues from the C-terminal of fibrin, which is essentially required for the binding of plasminogen to t-PA. This makes fibrin an ineffective co-factor, which lead to a decreased t-PA-mediated plasminogen activation. It also enhances the inhibition of plasmin by a_2-antiplasmin [15].

2.4 Diseases of the anticoagulant system (hypercoagulable states)

2.4.1 Virchow's triad

In 1845, the German physician, anthropologist, pathologist, prehistorian, and biologist, Rudolf Ludwig Carl Virchow hypothesised that three factors are important to the development of thrombosis; vascular endothelial injury, haemodynamic alterations and hypercoagulability, which interact with each other (**Figure 3**) [17]. The vascular endothelial injury was identified first as the main initiator of arterial thrombosis alongside traumatic or endocardial damaged. Moreover, the dysfunctional endothelial cells can secrete a significant concentration of procoagulant agents, including platelet adhesion molecules, TF, and PAI-1 while generating little anticoagulant effectors, such as TM and PCL [18]. The haemodynamic changes may promote procoagulant activities and leucocytic adhesions by modifying the gene expression of the endothelial cells. Although blood stasis is the main trigger for venous thrombosis, turbulent blood flow could also facilitate cardiac and arterial thrombosis. In hypercoagulability, blood clotting factors themselves facilitate thrombogenesis through heritable hypercoagulable states, such as mutations in Factor V Leiden (FVL) and prothrombin. Additionally, disseminated intravascular coagulopathy (DIC), heparin-mediated thrombocytopenia, and Trousseau's syndrome have been linked with hypercoagulability [18].

Hypercoagulability or thrombophilia defines a pathologic condition of exaggerated coagulation or coagulation without bleeding episode. It represents the increased risk for thrombose [19]. Hypercoagulability states are either acquired or inherited but real thrombosis originates as a result of interactions of both genetic and environmental agents. It encompasses a wide range of coagulation abnormalities characterised by a thrombotic event, such as deep vein thrombosis (DVT) and pulmonary embolism (PE). Congenital hypercoagulability included prothrombin G20210A gene mutation, deficiencies in protein C and protein S, AT deficiency and a single-point mutation on the FVL. Acquired conditions usually result from trauma or surgery, certain medications while the APS has been identified as the most common acquired thrombophilia in the general population [20]. The genetic abnormalities of the fibrinolytic system are not common, however, the acquired hyperfibrinolysis has been identified as the major cause of severe haemorrhage [15].

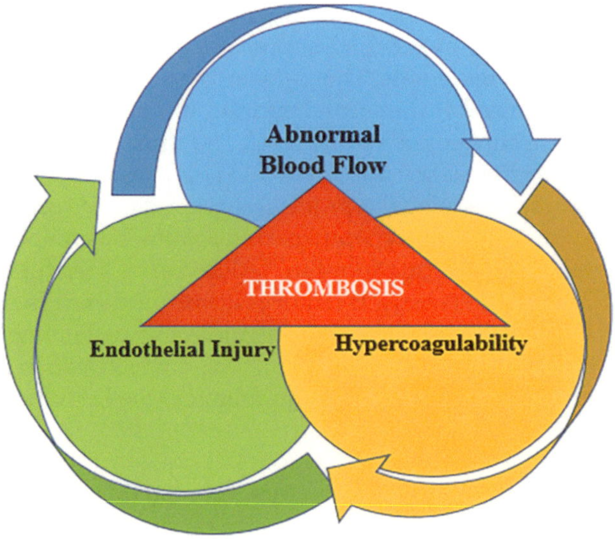

Figure 3.
Mechanisms of Virchow Triad in the Pathophysiology of Thrombus Formation: Rudolf Virchow proposed a triad of conditions that predisposes to thrombotic formation. They include abnormalities in the blood vessel wall, blood stasis and hypercoagulability. Inflammation, endothelial dysfunction, and atherosclerosis constituted abnormalities in the blood vessel wall. Abnormal blood flow arises from haemorheology and turbulence at bifurcations and stenotic sites. The hypercoagulability encompasses the abnormal blood constituents, including dysfunctional platelet, coagulation and endogenous fibrinolytic abnormalities, and metabolic factors.

2.4.2 Agents of hypercoagulability

Antithrombin III (ATIII) deficiency: ATIII inhibit coagulation by binding to heparin of the endothelial cells and forms a complex with thrombin [thrombin-antithrombin (TAT) complex]. The deficiency could manifest as an early age thrombosis and have the highest risk of thrombotic events among the hypercoagulable disorders. The incidence rate may be 1:500 in the general population. ATIII is produced in the liver independent of vitamin K. Its deficiency could occur because of decreased synthesis or increased loss, due to nephrotic syndrome, microangiopathy, and cardiopulmonary bypass surgery, enteropathy, DIC, sepsis, burn, and trauma [21]. Qualitative deficiency of ATIII, also known as a type-II deficiency, defines mutations that either involves the heparin-binding site (HBS), the reactive site (RS), leading to pleiotropic effects (PE), characterised by normal ATIII levels but with decreased activity [22].

Protein C and S deficiencies: Protein C and S deficiencies might be inherited but are sometimes inducible by some other conditions, including vitamin K antagonists, liver dysfunction, renal failure, DIC, and active thrombosis. Protein S promotes the activity of the enhanced protein C. The aetiology of acquired protein S defects are similar to acquired protein C deficiency, including warfarin therapy, liver cirrhosis, pregnancy, chronic disease and vitamin K deficiency. Protein C binds to TM and becomes APC. APC has been reported to exhibit anti-inflammatory, anticoagulant, and cytoprotective activities. It inactivates coagulation FV and VIII while FVL mutation is a major cause for APC resistance and the most prevalent genetic thrombophilia [22].

The FV Leiden mutation: Is the most frequent inherited risk factor for thrombophilia. The FV Leiden mutation is believed to increase the risk of arterial thrombosis. It increases the chance of thrombosis by facilitating the synthesis of thrombin [21].

The prothrombin G20210A mutation: Prothrombin also known as FII, is the precursor of thrombin, known to be associated with a single point mutation. The prothrombin G20210A mutation is the second inherited risk factor for thrombosis. It leads to increased levels of prothrombin that shows an increased risk for arterial and venous thrombotic events caused by a single point mutation [15].

Hyperhomocysteinemia is characterised by premature thrombosis initiated by defective methionine metabolic pathway. Deficiencies of vitamin B_6, B_{12}, folate or defective enzymes activities, including cystathionine beta-synthase (CBS) or methylenetetrahydrofolate reductase (MTHFR), inhibit the effects of homocysteine metabolism. Other factors, such as hypothyroidism, renal failure, certain medications, including methotrexate, phenytoin, and carbamazepine improve homocysteine levels [23].

Elevated factor VIII (FVIII) is associated with an increased chance of thrombosis. An ABO blood group O individuals present with the lower levels of FVIII. An increased concentration of FVIII is linked with APC resistance irrespective of FV mutation while its low levels correlate with haemophilia A patients bleeding [22].

The sticky platelet syndrome is an autosomal dominant disorder through which platelets interacts with epinephrine or adenosine diphosphate (ADP) to stimulate hypercoagulability [15].

Antiphospholipid syndrome (APS) is the common acquired thrombophilia in which the antibodies are directed against phospholipids of cell membranes. The conditions occur in 3%–5% of the general population and are associated with arterial and venous thrombosis, sometimes leading to foetal loss. The diagnosis of antiphospholipid antibodies (APLAs) included lupus anticoagulant (LA), anti-beta-2-glycoprotein and anticardiolipin that lead to the prolongation of coagulation (aPTT) [19].

The interrelationship between inflammation and the coagulation system: Inflammation promotes a hypercoagulable state. The activation of the complement system by endotoxin lead to thrombocytopenia and hypercoagulability. The association between inflammation and coagulation was demonstrated in subjects with vasculitis, septic thromboembolism and purpura [24]. While coagulation inhibits the accumulation of infection, certain bacteria utilise fibrinolytic activities to counteract the effects. For instance, autoimmune conditions, such as immune thrombocytopenic purpura, polyarteritis nodosa, polymyositis, dermatomyositis, systemic lupus erythematosus, dermatomyositis, inflammatory bowel disease, and Behcet's syndrome, all facilitate the progress to thrombotic events [25].

Disorders of the fibrinolytic system, including plasminogen, dysfibrinogenemia, t-PA and FXII deficiencies, which are involved in plasmin generation, as well as an increase in PAI levels. Plasminogen defects clinically have similar thrombin manifestation to protein C deficiency at an early age. Inherited conditions of the fibrinolytic system are uncommon, and when the deficiency resulted in a hyperfibrinolytic state, then it could lead to a bleeding episode. Mutations that suppress the fibrinolytic system could predispose to thromboembolic events [15].

Plasminogen deficiency: Type-1 plasminogen deficiency, termed hypoplasminogenaemia, is a quantitative abnormality associated with decreased amounts and activities of plasminogen, characterised by hydrocephalus and uncommon inherited conjunctivitis. Type II plasminogen deficiency, known as dysplasminogenaemia, attributed to decreased activities of plasminogen due to a malfunctioning plasminogen molecule [26].

PAI-1 deficiency: Inherited PAI-1 defect is uncommon and is characterised by mild-to-moderate bleeding aggravated by trauma or surgery. It is associated with certain conditions of menorrhagia [26]. High PAI-1 levels have been investigated in certain conditions, including coronary artery disease, obesity, hyperlipidaemia, diabetes mellitus, and might be associated with the increased chance of arterial thrombosis in these disorders [15].

α_2-Antiplasmin deficiency also termed as Miyasato disease, is an uncommon autosomal condition associated with bleeding episodes due to hyperfibrinolysis [12].

Dysfibrinogenaemia is a condition associated with the presence of abnormal FN. The symptoms might present either a bleeding tendency, a tendency to thrombosis or a predisposition to both bleeding and thrombosis. While inherited dysfibrinogenaemia is rarely seen, the acquired dysfibrinogenaemia might be present in certain conditions, including multiple myeloma, trauma patients, liver cirrhosis, amniotic fluid embolism, and conditions with an elevated synthesis of t-PA. This disorder could lead to DIC and severe haemorrhage [26].

Common acquired hypercoagulable states:

Smoking: Tobacco has been shown to contain several toxic compounds, including nicotine, which cause significant damage to endothelial cells. Tobacco smoke could inhibit the release of t-PA and TFPI while carbon monoxide promotes the permeability of lipid to the endothelium, which could further progress the formation of atheroma [19].

Trauma is the common type of is acquired hypercoagulable state. The imbalance between the procoagulant and anticoagulant agents is more pronounced within the first 24 hours of injury. The multiorgan failure due to respiratory distress syndrome following trauma has been linked with the increased TF levels [19].

Pregnancy: During pregnancy, the imbalance between the elevated procoagulants and the decrease in the anticoagulants, including t-PA, in addition to stasis are triggered by compression of the gravid uterus. Pregnancy increases the time of hypercoagulability during the postpartum period [27].

Heparin has been prescribed as an anticoagulant but under certain conditions, prolonged heparin administration has been reported to paradoxically cause arterial and venous thrombosis concomitantly with thrombocytopenia, known as "heparin-induced thrombocytopenia (HIT)" [19].

Endogenous and exogenous hormones influence coagulation: Existing reports have shown that oral contraception and hormone therapy could facilitate thrombosis, leading to cardiovascular events. Testosterone therapy has been implicated with thrombotic risk by increasing blood pressure, hyperviscosity, platelet aggregation, and haemoglobin cholesterol [28, 29].

Other acquired hypercoagulability states include:

- Certain medications, such as those prescribed to treat certain cancers, including thalidomide, tamoxifen, bevacizumab, and lenalidomide
- Central venous catheter placement, hyperlipidaemia, obesity
- Prolonged immobility, inactivity or bed rest
- Heart attacks, including cardiac heart failure, stroke pelvic artery diseases, etc.
- Long-distance aeroplane travel, known as "economy class syndrome"

- Previous history of DVT or PE
- Myeloproliferative, including polycythaemia vera or essential thrombocytosis
- Paroxysmal nocturnal haemoglobinuria
- Inflammatory bowel syndrome
- HIV/AIDS
- Nephrotic syndrome (too much protein in the urine).

2.5 Investigations of hypercoagulability

Hypercoagulability has been recognised as an abnormal complex condition of the haemostasis and as such, the diagnosis of hypercoagulability syndromes involves a combination of associated risk factors, screening tests and confirmation tests [21]. Assessment guidelines vary between medical associations. Some associations suggested that young patients with unprovoked or recurrent VTE, patients with a strong family history of abnormal blood clotting, patients with a recurrent blood clot, women with a history of recurrent miscarriage, stroke at a young age, thromboses in unusual sites, such as hepatic, renal, cerebral, mesenteric, neonatal purpura fulminans, warfarin-induced skin necrosis, and foetal loss should be screened for haemophilia. Also, patients with a history of suspected APS, unexplained prothrombin time (PT), thrombin time (TT), may require APS investigation, screening for APLAs and the diluted Russell venom viper test (dRVVT) [21].

The baseline investigations for hypercoagulability states, including routine coagulation studies, such as aPPT, which measures the blood clot time, usually to monitor heparin treatment, prothrombin time (PT) test is used to calculate INR, to monitor warfarin (Coumadin) treatment, FN levels, d-dimer and complete blood counts (CBC) should be carried out. The most advanced and essential screenings for thrombophilia include functional assays for ATIII, protein C and S deficiencies, PCR for prothrombin G2021A mutation and FVL mutation, testing for APLAs and homocysteine levels [19].

Screening for undetected cancer and unexplained VTE in older patients, including patients history and physical examination, ESR, hepatic and renal function tests, urinalysis, and chest X-ray (XR), tumour markers, CT of the chest, abdomen and pelvis mammography in women above 40 years [20], prostate ultrasound in men of more than 50 years, lower endoscopy, Papanicolaou smear and faecal occult blood test are recommended. In patients with hypercoagulability syndromes, there is an increased risk of venous thrombosis than ischemic stroke. Existing evidence has indicated that venous thrombosis could progress to arterial strokes by paradoxical embolism, therefore young adults with stroke should be screened for venous thrombosis, as the incidence of stroke is gradually increasing in young adults. The report has indicated an association between the homocystinuria and APLA syndrome with arterial strokes, and stroke has been investigated as the common arterial condition progressing to APLA syndrome. Hence, screening for APLA syndrome should be performed on stroke patients younger than 45 years [19].

2.5.1 Other tests to investigate acquired hypercoagulable states

Anticardiolipin antibodies (ACA) or beta-2 glycoproteins, LA, which are part of the APLA syndrome, to evaluate patients with recurrent miscarriage and venous or arterial thrombosis. Heparin antibodies (in patients who have decreased platelet counts after exposure to heparin) [19].

2.6 Management of hypercoagulability

Anticoagulant medications include synthetic drugs, including warfarin (Coumadin), which is taken orally, heparin, which is given either intravenously (IV), or subcutaneously. LMWH is injected also subcutaneously, fondaparinux (Arixtra) is also injected subcutaneously and are the most commonly prescribed drug available worldwide [19, 26].

The ATIII can be substituted for inherited or acquired defects, such as enhanced consumption in DIC and sepsis. Fresh frozen plasma (FFP) for the maintenance of natural balance between procoagulant and anticoagulant factors [30]. Also, various types of anticoagulants and antiplatelets are established to treat recurrent VTE [31], such as vitamin K antagonist (VKA), aspirin (as evaluated in the WARFASA and ASPIRE trials), rivaroxaban (EINSTEIN trial), dabigatran (RE-MEDY and RE-SONATE trials), and apixaban (AMPLIFY trial. The CLOT trial also evaluated LMWH against warfarin in cancer patients and was approved by food and drugs administration [32], rosuvastatin was approved for the prevention of occurrence of VTE [19].

3. Traditional medications

Although the present anticoagulant drugs available are safe and effective, the morbidity and mortality caused by atherothrombosis are still unacceptably high [33]. Many of these drugs are mostly associated with several side effects [34]. Statin, such as simvastatin, a lipid-lowering agent, known as 3-hydroxy-3-methyl-glutaryl coenzyme A reductase inhibitor, is associated with several side effects, including fever, headache, gastric irritation, myositis, hyperuricaemia, rhabdomyolysis, myalgia, renal and hepatic dysfunctions [35]. Acetylsalicylic acid, including aspirin, are antiplatelet synthetic drugs widely prescribed to treat inflammation, headache, fever and thrombosis [36]. Aspirin, in particular, has been reported to inhibit cyclooxygenase (COX), a potent enzyme that catalyses prostaglandin formation by blocking the synthesis of thromboxane A2 (TXA2), an essential mediator of blood clotting [37]. However, aspirin and other related antiplatelet drugs were reported to give recurrent thromboembolic vascular events (aspirin intolerance), including dizziness, nausea, abdominal pain or patients may suffer from increased risk of bleeding [37]. Bleeding is the most common complication associated with warfarin therapy and is related to exponentially higher INR values. The goal of the management is to reduce the INR back to a therapeutic safe level [13]. Existing reports have shown that plant extracts have analgesic, antioxidant, anti-inflammatory, anticoagulative, antiplatelet, anti-atherosclerotic, antithrombosis antiproliferative, and cardioprotective, properties [38, 39]. In this regard, the development of natural-based products to augment conventional synthetic drugs is essential. They are more effective with minimal or without side effects [40]. Some natural-based products commonly used in traditional medicines include:

Ginger (Zingiber officinale Roscoe) is a well-known natural Chinese herbal medicine, widely used to treat ailments, including gastrointestinal tract disorders, arthritis cardiomyopathy, high blood pressure and palpitations [41]. The main chemical compounds present in ginger include gingerol, shogaol, zingerone and paradol [42]. The 6-Gingerol has a lot of therapeutic potentials, including antioxidant, antitumor and anti-inflammatory effects [43, 44]. Previous report has demonstrated that ginger exhibit anti-atherothrombotic activity by suppressing platelet aggregation and TXB2 secretion in vitro. Previous study has shown that ginger crude extracts exhibit hypotensive, endothelium-independent vasodilatory and cardio-suppressive activities through their specific inhibitory action on voltage-dependent calcium channels [45].

Allium sativum (garlic): Plant extracts facilitate the treatment of atherosclerosis through various mechanisms of action at different pathways [46, 47]. The extracts from garlic have been demonstrated to show the most remarkable and clear cardio-protective activity since garlic can attenuate lipids profile through the inhibition of cholesterol biosynthesis, reduction of LDL, ameliorate arterial hypertension, and prevent platelet aggregation [48–50]. Therefore, garlic appears to be a promising plant for atherothrombotic treatment and prevention. The alliinase enzyme presence in garlic is well potentiated and have been used in the treatment of CVDs. The oxidative inhibitory phytochemicals present in garlic contribute significantly to improving the levels of HDL. The phytochemical contents of garlic also, including selenium, flavonoids, allixin, water and lipid-soluble organosulphur have been identified to regulate oxidative activities, while s-allylcysteine and other water-soluble chemicals of garlic are also found to be responsible for the anti-oxidant effects [38].

Citrus Limon (lemon): Over time, the prevalence of CVDs is grossly increasing. Flavonoids are very common plant natural-based products that have multiple therapeutic benefits and other biological functions [51]. The flavonoids contained in citrus included flavanones, flavones, and flavanols. Structurally, flavonoids could be categorised into six major classes, including flavanones, flavones, flavanols, isoflavones, flavonols, and anthocyanidins [52]. Flavonoids are polyphenol compounds associated with antioxidant activities, including inhibition of platelet activation and aggregation, anticancer, and anti-inflammatory activities since an increased dietary intake of antioxidants could prevent atherosclerosis, as increased cholesterol and occlusion is correlated. Structurally, flavonoids could be categorised into six major classes, including flavanones, flavones, flavanols, isoflavones, flavonols, and anthocyanidins [52]. Even though the flavones and flavanols are in low concentrations compared to flavanones, but are more potent antioxidants and free radical scavengers [53]. The high contents of phytochemicals, including naringin, hesperidin, limonene, and other flavonoids in citrus limon could significantly reduce the morbidity or mortality in the patients at risk of developing cardiovascular events [53].

Malus Domestica (apple) apple cider vinegar (ACV): The chemical constituents available in apple include catechin, caffeic acid, gallic acid, chlorogenic acids and p-coumaric acid have been demonstrated to show high antioxidant potential. Apples have high nutritional value and are important source of several phytochemicals, including phenolic compounds, flavonoids, organic acids, minerals and vitamins, minerals, calcium, potassium, phosphorus and low acetic acid, which have been useful for many years in the treatment of various metabolic conditions [54]. Previous study has indicated that ACV exerts its therapeutic effects by improving atherogenesis, attenuating inflammatory responses and reducing triacylglycerol as observed in mice serum [55]. Dietary flavonoids extracted from apples decreased the levels of inflammation associated biomarkers, such as IL-11 and IL-2 in the intestine of mice [56]. The phytochemicals present in apples, such as polyphenols, polysaccharides, sterols, and triterpenes, jointly contributed to its antioxidants, anti-cancer, and anti-inflammatory activities, such as anti-inflammatory, anticancer and inhibition of platelet activation [57].

Honey: A multi-nutrient food comprising different quantities of minerals, such as aluminium, barium, boron, chlorine, fluoride, iodine, sulphur and potassium, which account for one-third of the total elements [58, 59]. Honey has been demonstrated to contain polyphenols compounds, mostly flavonoids, phenolic acids, and phenolic acid products, which have been reported to contribute greatly to its antioxidant activities [60]. It is naturally produced by bees and is mainly obtained from flowering plants. Honey is divided into two categories; nectar honey, originating from plant nectars, and honeydew honey, mainly secreted by plant-sucking insects (Hemiptera) [61]. Previous results indicated that honey-mediated, inhibition of platelet aggregation, prolongation of aPTT, PT, and TT and reduction in FN levels. The mechanism by which honey inhibits platelet aggregation can be explained by the amount of hydrogen peroxide present in honey. Reports have shown that exogenous exposure to hydrogen peroxide led to platelet inhibition and therefore, it could be hypothesised that the presence of hydrogen peroxide might be the primary basis of honey induced inhibition of platelet aggregation [62]. Moreover, natural honey is known to have suppressive potentials on reactive oxygen species, pinpointing that activated platelets could release various cytokines which in turn might activate phagocytes. Therefore, platelet activated phagocytes lead to an increase in the synthesis of free oxygen radicals. Because honey inhibits platelet aggregation, it is suggested that honey could indirectly suppress the generation of free oxygen radicals. Remarkably, free oxygen radicals have been reported to act on platelet activity through oxidative modification of lipids and their derivatives and hence, it could be proposed that honey might promote platelet function by suppressing LDL oxidation, which could indirectly affect platelet function [63].

Existing reports demonstrate that honey inhibited the coagulation proteins of the three coagulation pathways: intrinsic, extrinsic, and final common pathway. The main reason for the anticoagulant properties of nature might be attributed to the variety of flavonoids contained in honey that may affect the activity of coagulation factors like FN and factor VII. Additionally, honey contains maltose that has been reported to interfere with blood coagulation. The therapeutic potentials of honey comprise various mechanisms that might play a significant role in the prevention of atherosclerotic CVDs. Honey has been reported to inhibit thrombin (main enzyme of blood coagulation) and induce the formation of reactive oxygen species from phagocytes; as free oxygen radicals particularly superoxide and hypochlorous acid provides room for the development of atherosclerotic plaque, thus honey might interrupt the formation of atherosclerotic plaque [62].

4. Conclusion

The anticoagulant mechanisms maintain the constant blood flow while inhibiting the progress to hypercoagulable states. The process of maintaining the delicate balance between the coagulation system, the integrity of the haemostasis and the significant contributions of the various system involved is continuous. Supplementation with traditional medications could be beneficial in the treatment and prevention of hypercoagulable states. Further studies are required to evaluate the new classes of anticoagulants and traditional medications with anticoagulant potentials towards improving healthcare to the patients demanding hypercoagulable therapy.

DOI: http://dx.doi.org/10.5772/intechopen.103774

Author details

Ibrahim Kalle Kwaifa
Department of Haematology, School of Medical Laboratory Sciences, College of Health Sciences, Usmanu Danfodiyo University (UDU), Sokoto, Nigeria

*Address all correspondence to: nanamarye2009@gmail.com

References

[1] Scott CH, Hassan M & Yaish MD. Pediatric Thromboembolism eMedicine. https://emedicine.medscape.com/article/959501-print

[2] Vilahur G, Ben-Aicha S, Badimon L. New insights into the role of adipose tissue in thrombosis. Cardiovascular Research. July 2017;**113**(9):1046-1054. DOI: 10.1093/cvr/cvx086

[3] Bagoly Z, Koncz Z, Hársfalvi J, Muszbek L. Factor XIII, clot structure, thrombosis. Thrombosis Research. 2012;**129**:382-387

[4] Cristina M, Sena CM, Fernanda C, Seiça RM. Endothelial Dysfunction in Type 2 Diabetes: Targeting Inflammation. We are IntechOpen, the world's Lead Publ Open Access books Built by Sci, Sci TOP 1% 2018. DOI: 105772/intechopen76994

[5] Segovia SA, Vickers MH, Gray C, Reynolds CM. Maternal obesity, inflammation, and developmental programming. BioMed Research International. 2014;**2014**:418975. DOI: 10.1155/2014/418975

[6] Segovia SA, Vickers MH, Reynolds CM. The impact of maternal obesity on inflammatory processes and consequences for later offspring health outcomes. Journal of Developmental Origins of Health and Disease. 2019;**8**:529-540

[7] Papapanagiotou A, Siasos G, Kassi E, Gargalionis AN, Papavassiliou AG. Novel inflammatory markers in hyperlipidaemia: Clinical implications. Current Medicinal Chemistry. 2015;**22**:2727-2743

[8] Katakami N. Mechanism of development of atherosclerosis and cardiovascular disease in diabetes mellitus. Journal of Atherosclerosis and Thrombosis. 1 Jan 2018;**25**(1):27-39. DOI: 10.5551/jat.RV17014

[9] Barale C, Russo I. Influence of cardiometabolic risk factors on platelet function. International Journal of Molecular Sciences. 2020;**21**(2):623. DOI: 10.3390/ijms21020623

[10] Badimon L, Padró T, Vilahur G. Atherosclerosis, platelets and thrombosis in acute ischaemic heart disease. European Heart Journal Acute Cardiovascular Care. 2012;**1**:60-74

[11] Barrachina MN, Sueiro AM, Izquierdo I, Hermida-Nogueira L, Guitián E, Casanueva FF, et al. GPVI surface expression and signalling pathway activation are increased in platelets from obese patients: Elucidating potential anti-atherothrombotic targets in obesity. Atherosclerosis. 2019;**2019**(281):62-70

[12] Umerah CO, Momodu II. Anticoagulation. [Updated 2021 Dec 27]. In: StatPearls [Internet]. Treasure Island (FL): StatPearls Publishing; Jan 2022

[13] Falk E, Fuster V. Atherothrombosis: Disease burden, activity, and vulnerability. In: Fuster V, Harrington RA, Narula J, Eapen ZJ, editors. Hurst's The Heart, 14e. McGraw Hill; 2017. Available from: https://accessmedicine.mhmedical.com/content.aspx?bookid=2046&sectionid=176555141 [Accessed March 14, 2022]

[14] Barr D, Epps QJ. Direct oral anticoagulants: A review of common medication errors. Journal of Thrombosis and Thrombolysis. 2019;**47**:146-154

[15] Frca JAE, Frca NH. Anticlotting mechanisms 1: Physiology and pathology. 2013;**13**:87-92

[16] Rijken DC, Lijnen HR. New insights into the molecular mechanisms of the fibrinolytic system. Journal of Thrombosis and Haemostasis. 2009;7:4-13

[17] Hashimoto H, Usui G, Tsugeno Y, et al. Cerebral thromboembolism after lobectomy for lung cancer: Pathological diagnosis and mechanism of thrombus formation. Cancers (Basel). 2019;**11**:1-17

[18] Xu S, Bendeck M, Gotlieb A. Vascular pathobiology: Atherosclerosis and large vessel disease. In: Buja LM, Bot J, editors. Cardiovasc Pathology. 4th ed. The Netherlands: Elsevier Amsterdam; 2016. pp. 85-124

[19] Senst B, Tadi P, Goyal A. Hypercoagulability Pathophysiology. statpearl Publ NCBI Bokkshelf 2021; pp. 1-10

[20] Dawood F, Andrea T. Inherited and Acquired Thrombophilia in Pregnancy. Rijeka: Intechopen; 2011. ISBN: 978-953-307-872-4, http://www.intechopen.co

[21] Nakashima MO, Rogers HJ. Hypercoagulable states: An algorithmic approach to laboratory testing and update on monitoring of direct oral anticoagulants. Blood Research. 2014;**49**:85-94

[22] Saint S, Chopra V. The Saint-Chopra Guide to Inpatient Medicine. 4 ed. Oxford, UK: Oxford University Press; 2018. Available from: https://oxfordmedicine.com/view/10.1093/med/9780190862800.001.0001/med-9780190862800

[23] Lima LG, Monteiro RQ. Activation of blood coagulation in cancer: Implications for tumour progression. Bioscience Reports. 2013;**33**(5):e00064. DOI: 10.1042/BSR20130057

[24] Emmi G, Silvestri E, Squatrito D, Amedei A, Niccolai E, D'Elios MM, et al. Thrombosis in vasculitis: From pathogenesis to treatment. Thrombosis Journal. 16 Apr 2015;**13**:15. DOI: 10.1186/s12959-015-0047-z

[25] Tamaki H, Khasnis A. Venous thromboembolism in systemic autoimmune diseases: A narrative review with emphasis on primary systemic vasculitides. Vascular Medicine. 2015;**20**:369-370

[26] Chapin JC, Hajjar KA. Fibrinolysis and the control of blood coagulation. Blood Reviews. 2015;**29**(1):17-24. DOI: 10.1016/j.blre.2014.09.003

[27] Kahn SR, Lim W, Dunn AS, et al. Prevention of VTE in nonsurgical patients: Antithrombotic therapy and prevention of thrombosis, 9th ed: American College of Chest Physicians Evidence-Based Clinical Practice Guidelines. Chest. 2012;**141**: e1955-e2265

[28] Freedman J, Glueck CJ, Prince M, Riaz R, Wang P. Testosterone, thrombophilia, thrombosis. Translational Research. 2015;**165**:537-548

[29] Glueck CJ, Richardson-Royer C, Schultz R, Burger T, Bowe D, Padda J, et al. Testosterone therapy, thrombophilia-hypofibrinolysis, and hospitalization for deep venous thrombosis-pulmonary embolus: An exploratory, hypothesis-generating study. Clinical and Applied Thrombosis/Hemostasis. 2014;**20**:244-248

[30] Stevens SM, Woller SC, Bauer KA, Kasthuri R, Cushman M, Streiff M, et al. Guidance for the evaluation and treatment of hereditary and acquired thrombophilia. Journal of Thrombosis and Thrombolysis. 2016;**41**:154-164

[31] Barnes GD, Kanthi Y, Froehlich JB. Venous thromboembolism: Predicting recurrence and the need for extended anticoagulation. Vascular Medicine. 2015;**20**:143-152

[32] Ormesher L, Simcox L, Tower C, Greer IA. Management of inherited thrombophilia in pregnancy. Womens Heal (Lond). 2016;**12**:433-441

[33] Dias S, Paredes S, Ribeiro L. Drugs involved in dyslipidemia and obesity treatment: Focus on adipose tissue. International Journal of Endocrinology. 2018:2637418. DOI: 10.1155/2018/2637418

[34] Khan SJ, Afroz S, Khan RA. Antihyperlipidemic and anti-hyperglycemic effects of Cymbopogon jwarancusa in high-fat high-sugar diet model. Pakistan Journal of Pharmaceutical Sciences. 2018;**31**:1341-1345

[35] Hussain MS, Jahan N, Or Rashid MM, et al. Antihyperlipidemic screening and plasma uric acid reducing potential of *Momordica charantia* seeds on Swiss albino mice model. Heliyon. 2019;**5**:e01739

[36] Qadir MI, Manzoor A, Akash MSH. Potential role of medicinal plants for anti-atherosclerosis activity. Bangladesh Journal of Pharmacology. 2018;**13**:59-66

[37] Karam I, Ma N, Liu XW, Li JY, Yang YJ. Effect of aspirin on hyperlipidemia in rats. JSM Pharmacology and Clinical Toxicology. 2019;**2019**(1):6

[38] Kirichenko TV, Sukhorukov VN, Markin AM, et al. Medicinal plants as a potential and successful treatment option in the context of atherosclerosis. Frontiers in Pharmacology. 2020;**11**:1-15

[39] Wlosinska M, Nilsson AC, Hlebowicz J, Hauggaard A, Kjellin M, Fakhro M, et al. The effect of aged garlic extract on the atherosclerotic process – a randomized double-blind placebo-controlled trial. BMC Complementary Medicine and Therapies. 2020;**20**:132. DOI: 10.1186/s12906-020-02932-5

[40] Newman DJ, Cragg GM. Natural products as sources of new drugs from 1981 to 2014. Journal of Natural Products. 2016;**79**:629-661

[41] Baliga MS, Haniadka R, Pereira MM, Thilakchand KR, Rao S, Arora A. Radioprotective effects of Zingiber officinale roscoe (ginger): Past, present and future. Food & Function. 2012;**3**:714-723

[42] Wu HC, Horng CT, Tsai SC, et al. Relaxant and vasoprotective effects of ginger extracts on porcine coronary arteries. International Journal of Molecular Medicine. 2018;**41**:2420-2428

[43] Mashhadi NS, Ghiasvand R, Askari G, Hariri M, Darvishi L, Mofid MR. Anti-oxidative and anti-inflammatory effects of ginger in health and physical activity: Review of current evidence. International Journal of Preventive Medicine. 2013;**4**:S36-S42

[44] Weng CJ, Chou CP, Ho CT, Yen GC. Molecular mechanism inhibiting human hepatocarcinoma cell invasion by 6-shogaol and 6-gingerol. Molecular Nutrition & Food Research. 2012;**56**:1304-1314

[45] Gilani AH, Mandukhail SU, Iqbal J, Yasinzai M, Aziz N, Khan A, et al. Antispasmodic and vasodilator activities of Morinda citrifolia root extract are mediated through blockade of voltage dependent calcium channels. BMC Complementary and Alternative Medicine. 2010;**10**:2

[46] El-Zayat MM, Eraqi MM, Alrefai H, et al. The antimicrobial, antioxidant,

and anticancer activity of greenly synthesized selenium and zinc composite nanoparticles using Ephedra aphylla extract. Biomolecules. 2021;**11**:470

[47] Karagodin VP, Sobenin IA, Orekhov AN. Antiatherosclerotic and cardioprotective effects of time-released garlic powder pills. Current Pharmaceutical Design. 2016;**2017**(22):196-213. DOI: 10.2174/138 1612822666151112153351

[48] Sedaghat A, Shahbazian H, Rezazadeh A, Haidari F, Jahanshahi A, Mahmoud Latifi S, et al. The effect of soy nut on serum total antioxidant, endothelial function and cardiovascular risk factors in patients with type 2 diabetes. Diabetes and Metabolic Syndrome: Clinical Research and Reviews. 2019;**13**:1387-1391. DOI: 10.1016/ j.dsx.2019.01.057

[49] Adab Z, Eghtesadi S, Vafa MR, Heydari I, Shojaii A, Haqqani H, et al. Effect of turmeric on glycemic status, lipid profile, hs-CRP, and total antioxidant capacity in hyperlipidemic type 2 diabetes mellitus patients. Phytotherapy Research. 2019;**33**:1173-1181. DOI: 10.1002/ptr.6312

[50] Xu C, Mathews AE, Rodrigues C, Eudy BJ, Rowe CA, O'Donoughue A, et al. Aged garlic extract supplementation modifies inflammation and immunity of adults with obesity: A randomized, double-blind, placebo-controlled clinical trial. Clinical Nutrition ESPEN. 2018;**24**:148-155. DOI: 10.1016/ j.clnesp.2017.11.01

[51] Mas-Capdevila A, Teichenne J, Domenech-Coca C, Caimari A, Del Bas JM, Escoté X, et al. Effect of hesperidin on cardiovascular disease risk factors: The role of intestinal microbiota on hesperidin bioavailability. Nutrients. 2020;**12**(5):1488. DOI: 10.3390/ nu12051488

[52] Mahmoud AM, Mohammed HM, Khadrawy SM, Galaly SR. Hesperidin protects against chemically induced hepatocarcinogenesis via modulation of Nrf2/ARE/HO-1, PPARγ and TGF-β1/ Smad3 signalling, and amelioration of oxidative stress and inflammation. Chemico-Biological Interactions. 2017;**277**:146-158

[53] Mallick N, Khan RA, Riaz A, Afroz S. Anticoagulant, antiplatelet and antianemic effects of citrus paradisi (grape fruit) juice in rabbits. Pharmacology & Pharmacy. 2016;7(10):397-406

[54] Tripathi S, Mazumder PM. Apple cider vinegar (ACV) and their pharmacological approach towards Alzheimer's disease (AD): A review. Indian Journal of Pharmaceutical Education and Research. 2020;**54**: S67-S74

[55] Wu Z, Xia Z, Wu B, Wei F, Lv X, Xie Y, et al. Lipid profiling in serum from apolipoprotein E-knock out mice fed with different diets and its application to the study of the regulatory effect on lipid metabolism. Food & Function. 2018;**9**:5103-5114

[56] Espley RV, Butts CA, Laing WA, Martell S, Smith H, McGhie TK, et al. Dietary flavonoids from modified apple reduce inflammation markers and modulate gut microbiota in mice. The Journal of Nutrition. 2014;**144**:146-154

[57] Starowicz M, Achrem-Achremowicz B, Piskuła MK, et al. Phenolic compounds from apples: Reviewing their occurrence, absorption, bioavailability, processing, and antioxidant activity - a review. Polish Journal of Food and Nutrition Sciences. 2020;**70**:321-336

[58] Cianciosi D, Forbes-Hernández TY, Afrin S, et al. Phenolic compounds

in honey and their associated health benefits: A review. Molecules. 2018;**23**:pii:E2322. DOI: 10.3390/molecules23092322

[59] Rahman M, Gan SH, Khalil MI. Neurological effects of honey: Current and future prospects. Evidence-based Complementary and Alternative Medicine. 2014;**2014**:958721. DOI: 10.1155/2014/958721

[60] Prasetyo RH, Safitri E. Effect of honey to mobilize endogenous stem cells in efforts intestinal and ovarian tissue regeneration in rats with protein-energy malnutrition. Asian Pacific Journal of Reproduction. 2016;**5**:198-203. DOI: 10.1016/j.apjr.2016.04.0

[61] Ramli NZ, Chin KY, Zarkasi KA, Ahmad F. A Review on the protective effects of honey against metabolic syndrome. Nutrients. 2018;**10**(8):1009. DOI: 10.3390/nu10081009

[62] Ahmed A, Khan RA, Azim MK, et al. Effect of natural honey on human platelets and blood coagulation proteins. Pakistan Journal of Pharmaceutical Sciences. 2011;**24**:389-397

[63] Ahmed S, Shah P, Ahmed O. Biochemistry, lipids. [Updated 2021 May 9]. In: Stat Pearls [Internet]. Treasure Island (FL): Stat Pearls Publishing; 2021

Chapter 2

Anticoagulation in Thrombophilia

Iris Bararu Bojan, Stefan Dobreanu, Oana Viola Badulescu, Maria Cristina Vladeanu, Andrei Bojan, Carmen Elena Plesoianu and Manuela Ciocoiu

Abstract

Thrombophilia is a condition of hypercoagulability, which is defined as an abnormality of blood clotting, disturbing the balance between procoagulants and anticoagulants in favor of the former, thus increasing the risk of thrombosis. It can be classified into different categories, such as genetic/administered; primary/secondary; permanent/transient; low risk/high risk. Venous thromboembolism is the main and most common complication of a hypercoagulable condition, with an enormous impact on any national health system. The pathophysiological mechanisms involved are at various stages of research, some of which are far from being fully elucidated. Treatment of thrombophilia differs—while most conditions do not require anticoagulation as primary prophylaxis, secondary prophylaxis may require transient or permanent anticoagulation. Treatment options include parenteral unfractionated heparin, low molecular weight heparin (LMWH), fondaparinux or orally administered vitamin K antagonists, and direct oral anticoagulants (DOAC), such as rivaroxaban, apixaban, dabigatran, with increasing indications as data accumulate from recent and ongoing studies and trials.

Keywords: thrombophilia, hypercoagulability, thromboembolism, anticoagulation, prophylaxis

1. Introduction

Clotting is a physiological property of the body to form clots and thus minimize blood loss at the site of injury. Normal blood flow is kept in balance by factors that promote clotting and by antithrombotic factors. A hypercoagulable state, which may be complicated by the development of thromboembolism, is a consequence of hyperactivity of clotting promoters or anticoagulant deficiency. But the interaction between the two facets is much more complex than this, as thrombosis can be influenced by the qualitative and quantitative properties of factors, for example, their secretion, accumulation, or degradation [1].

What Virchow described in 1856 as the triad of conditions that must be met to develop venous thrombosis is accepted nowadays as hypercoagulability, vascular stasis and vascular trauma underlie the pathophysiological mechanism that explains this situation. Arterial thrombosis, on the other hand, results from the rupture of an atherosclerotic plaque, which pierces the vascular endothelium, resulting in the formation of platelet-rich thrombus around it [1].

Thrombophilia is a hypercoagulable or prothrombotic state, which is defined as an abnormality of blood clotting, thus increasing the risk of thrombosis. It can be classified into different categories, depending on its mechanism of action, how it occurs, whether it is an acquired or an inborn disease. [Genetic vs. acquired; primary vs. secondary; permanent vs. transient; low risk vs. high risk].

The known possible causes of thrombophilia are listed in **Table 1** [3].

Type 1 or major thrombophilias are a group of rare diseases that include antithrombin deficiency, protein C deficiency, or protein S deficiency, which together occur in less than 1% of the population but account for up to 7% of patients with thrombosis [4].

Type 2 thrombophilias or minor thrombophilias are much more common, the most important example being the factor V Leiden mutation, which can be identified in 5% of the European-born population and 30–50% of patients referred for thrombophilia testing.

The prothrombin mutation affects 1–4% of the general population but is found in up to 15% of patients tested for thrombophilia. Both types of mutations are much more common in Caucasians and almost never found in patients of Asian or African descent [4].

Hereditary thrombophilias are those in which a genetic mutation inherited from one or both parents leads to a condition in which the function of certain proteins of the clotting system is impaired. The condition can be expressed as a deficiency or loss

Primary (genetic)	Secondary (acquired)
Factor V mutation (G1691A mutation; factor V Leiden)	Prolonged bed rest or immobilization
Prothrombin mutation (G20210A)	Myocardial infarction
5,10-Methylene tetrahydrofolate reductase (hyperhomocysteinemia)	Atrial fibrillation
Increased levels of factor VIII, IX, XI, or fibrinogen	Tissue injury (surgery, fracture, burn)
Antithrombin III deficiency	Cancer
Protein C deficiency	Prosthetic cardiac valves
Protein S deficiency	Disseminated intravascular coagulation
Fibrinolysis defect	Heparin-induced thrombocytopenia
Homozygous homocystinuria (deficiency of cystathionine B-synthase)	Antiphospholipid syndrome
	Cardiomyopathy
	Nephrotic syndrome
	Hyperestrogenic states (pregnancy and postpartum)
	Oral contraceptive use
	Sickle cell anemia
	Smoking
	Infection (Covid 19)

Table 1.
Thrombophilia causes, Robbins and Cotran pathologic basis of disease (ninth edition.) [2].

of function, best exemplified by mutations in the antithrombin, protein C, or protein S genes, or as a gain of function, such as mutations in factor V Leiden and prothrombin 20,210 A/G. Other conditions, although less common, are the presence of abnormal levels of clotting factors, elevated homocysteine, or defects in the fibrinolytic pathway. Nowadays, we have reached a point where gene factors can be identified in up to 30% of patients with thrombophilia [5, 6].

Acquired thrombophilia is a hypercoagulable status composed of the association of a divergent group of clinical conditions, which include malignancy, pregnancy, prolonged bed rest, postoperative, nephrotic syndrome, or lifestyle risk factors, such as smoking or obesity. But the most important example is an antiphospholipid syndrome which is also included in the guidelines and should be tested for each time thrombophilia is suspected [5].

Although hypercoagulability disorders are classified as either inherited or acquired, thrombosis develops due to the interaction of both genetic and environmental factors, which has led to the development of the multiple-hit hypothesis, thus providing a possible explanation for the differences observed between subjects carrying the same gene mutation [6].

In an article by R H Thomas, the CALMSHAPES mnemonic was proposed to more easily recall the different etiologies of the hypercoagulable state, which are as follows:

- Protein C deficiency
- Antiphospholipid syndrome
- Factor V Leiden mutation
- Malignancy

Syndrome	% in the general population	% in patients with venous thromboembolism	Relative risk of thromboembolism
Factor V Leiden (G1691A)	0.05–4.8	18.8	4
Factor V Leiden (A1691A)	0.02	1.5	80
Prothrombin G20210A	0.06–2.7	7.1	2.8
Low protein C levels	0.2–0.4	3.7	6.5
Low protein S levels	0.16–0.1	2.3	5.0
Low antithrombin levels	0.02	1.9	20
Hyperhomocysteinemia	5–7	10	2.95
High factor VIII levels	11	25	4.8
High factor IX levels	10	20	2.8
High factor XI levels	10	19	2.2
Lipoprotein (a)	7	20	3.2
Antiphospholipid antibody	0–7	5–15	5.5

Table 2.
Prevalence of different thrombophilias and the risk of developing venous thromboembolism [3].

- Protein S deficiency
- Hyperhomocysteinemia
- Antithrombin III deficiency
- Prothrombin G2021A mutation
- Factor eight excesses
- Sticky platelet syndrome [6]

Venous thromboembolism is the main and most common complication of a hypercoagulable condition, with a huge impact on any national health system. Available data from the United States estimates that venous thromboembolism is responsible for more than half a million hospitalizations annually, with an estimated cost of treatment per patient of more than $56,000, totaling an estimated $5–$20 billion. The different mechanisms of occurrence of a hypercoagulable state have different penetration in the general population, with different risk rates for complications, such as venous thromboembolism, as shown in **Table 2**.

2. Pathophysiology

2.1 Factor V Leiden

Factor V Leiden is an autosomal dominant transmissible gene abnormality that shows incomplete penetrance; therefore, the disease will not be developed by all carriers of the mutation. In terms of pathophysiological mechanism, factor V Leiden is also known as factor V Arg506Gln and as factor V R506Q, due to a single mutation of the factor V gene in which guanine replaces arginine at nucleotide 1691. Consequently, just one amino acid change, replacing arginine with glutamine, suppresses the binding site to the activated proteolytic protein C of factors V and Va [7, 8]. With the malformed binding site, the natural anticoagulant protein C can no longer bind and cleave factor V and Va to inactivate it, therefore factor V concentration increases and disrupts the pro−/anticoagulant balance, leading to an increased risk of thrombosis [7]. The result of the so-called activated protein C resistance phenotype is blamed in up to 95% of cases as a consequence of a factor V mutation, which has resulted in a 7-fold increase in the relative risk of developing deep vein thrombosis in patients [8].

2.2 Prothrombin G20210A

Prothrombin G20210A is a specific genetic mutation of nucleotide 20210A of the second factor of the coagulation cascade (factor II—prothrombin) and consists of a change of guanine to adenine, with a higher concentration of prothrombin found in mutation carriers [9]. Although several attempts have been made to explain why this happens, the exact mechanism of how the mutation leads to increased protein production, thereby increasing the overall risk of thrombosis, is not yet fully understood [10]. Caucasians have a higher risk of developing this condition, but the risk of thrombosis is minimal for heterozygotes in whom no other risk factors are identified.

However, in the presence of other secondary risk factors, such as prolonged bed rest or pregnancy, the risk is greatly increased. Homozygous carriers face an increased risk of thrombosis by 2 to 3 folds [11].

2.3 Protein C

Protein C and its activated form are vitamin K-dependent zymogens with an important role in the regulation of anticoagulation by inactivating coagulation factors Va and VIIIa [12].

Protein C deficiency is a rare abnormality that alters the activity of protein C, a consequence of which is the loss of activated protein C function and, consequently, its inability to control coagulation [13].

Mutations in the PROC gene are responsible for the development of congenital protein C deficiency and are transmitted in an autosomal dominant manner, affecting heterozygous carriers much less than homozygous carriers. To date, more than 160 PROC mutations have been identified, which can affect protein C concentration (type I) or result in the production of an altered protein with reduced activity and ineffective anticoagulant function (type II) [13].

Protein C is activated by interactions with thrombin after the latter has attached to thrombomodulin expressed on the endothelial cell surface. Activated protein C then proceeds to reduce clotting by cleaving and inactivating clotting factors Va and VIIIa. Low concentrations or structural alterations of protein C disturb the coagulation balance, favoring the development of a hypercoagulable state [13].

2.4 Protein S

Protein S is a vitamin K-dependent glycoprotein synthesized by the liver with an important role in coagulation, where it acts as a cofactor for protein C to inactivate coagulation factors Va and VIIIa and also as a cofactor for tissue factor pathway inhibitory protein, leading to inactivation of factor Xa and tissue factor/factor VII. In the human body, protein S exists in two forms—one free and one bound to the complementary protein C4b [13, 14].

Protein S deficiency is an unusual condition caused by quantitative or qualitative abnormalities following point mutations in the PROS1 gene. Mutations are transmitted in an autosomal dominant manner with incomplete penetrance. Homozygous individuals have a higher risk of thrombosis than heterozygous individuals, of whom only an estimated 50% develop venous thromboembolism, the other half remaining asymptomatic. More than 200 genetic mutations have been identified, causing a range of defects, which can be classified into three types—type I is characterized by low levels of total S protein and free S protein, type II total S protein concentrations are normal but with low activity, while type III has normal levels of total S protein but low levels of free S protein [13].

A quantitative or qualitative deficiency of protein S will have great implications in the regulation of coagulation, as the natural anticoagulant mechanisms will be less effective in inactivating coagulation factors Va, VIIIa, and VIIa, thus favoring a thrombosis-prone state.

2.5 Antiphospholipid syndrome

Antiphospholipid syndrome is an autoimmune-generated hypercoagulable state caused by the presence of antiphospholipid antibodies and is the most common cause of acquired thrombophilia. It is characterized by the presence of at least one of three antiphospholipid antibodies, which are lupus anticoagulant, anticardiolipin antibodies, or antibeta2 glycoprotein antibodies, in addition to one or more clinical manifestations of thrombosis [15, 16].

The condition can be classified into a primary antiphospholipid syndrome, which occurs without a concurrent autoimmune disease, and a secondary antiphospholipid syndrome, in the presence of another autoimmune condition, the most prominent example being systemic lupus erythematosus [15].

Two profile risks for thrombosis have been identified in terms of the type and titer of antibodies present:

A high-risk profile involves one of the following: Thromboembolism risk profile:

- the presence of lupus anticoagulant at 2 different measurements taken at least 12 weeks apart;
- any combination of 2 of the 3 defining antibodies;
- identification of all 3 antiphospholipid antibodies;
- the persistence of high antiphospholipid antibody titers;

A low-risk profile requires transient isolation of anticardiolipin antibodies or antibeta2 glycoprotein antibodies at low-to-medium titers [16].

The mechanisms involved in the generation of hypercoagulability require further investigation, as the few proposed mechanisms cannot exclusively explain this condition. Antiphospholipid antibodies are thought to interfere with platelet and endothelial cell membranes, proteins in the coagulation cascade or inhibit protein C.

The types, isotypes, and titers of antibodies found to correlate directly with the risk of thrombosis risk increases with higher titers, the presence of IgG antibodies, or the identification of lupus anticoagulant [15].

2.6 Malignancy

Thromboembolic complications in cancer patients are the second leading cause of mortality, presenting in various forms from venous or arterial thrombosis to disseminated intravascular coagulation. Venous thromboembolism is a significant cause of morbidity and mortality, with pulmonary embolism being three times more common than in a person who has developed venous thrombosis but does not have cancer [17, 18].

Other rarer thrombotic complications are also seen more frequently in patients with cancer, such as disseminated intravascular coagulation and thrombotic microangiopathy. Disseminated intravascular coagulation is a condition in which the coagulation cascade is activated systemically, resulting on the one hand in the formation of fibrin deposits that move to different organs blocking microcirculation, and on the other hand consuming clotting factors and platelets, which can lead to life-threatening bleeding [17, 19].

It has long been observed that patients with cancer and thromboembolic disease are strongly associated, but despite this, the mechanisms leading to the hypercoagulable state are numerous, complex, and not yet fully understood. Tumor-specific factors are also thought to play a role, because of the variable risk of thrombosis for different cancers. Returning to Virchow's triad, all three conditions for thrombosis can occur simultaneously in a cancer patient, the best example being venous stasis following venous compression by a tumor [17, 18].

Various cancer therapies can also contribute to a prothrombotic state, with many reports suggesting an association between chemotherapy and arterial thrombosis. The most implicated agents are platinum-based therapeutics (cisplatin) and those that interfere with vascular endothelial growth factor, either to inhibit it directly (bevacizumab) or to inhibit its receptor tyrosine kinase (sorafenib) [20].

2.7 Pregnancy

The hypercoagulable state observed during pregnancy is the result of physiological, hormonal, and physical changes that affect women during pregnancy and in the peri- and post-natal periods.

As a result of hormonal changes, levels of certain clotting factors are increased, such as those of factors VII, VIII, X, von Willebrand factor, and fibrinogen. Meanwhile, during the second and third trimesters, resistance to activated protein C has been observed, as well as decreased activity of protein S. The number of studies has also reported decreased activity of the fibrinolytic pathway, due to an increase in its inhibitors, such as plasminogen activator inhibitor 1 and 2 and activable fibrinolytic inhibitor. All of these changes contribute to a tilting of the coagulation balance toward a prothrombotic state [21, 22].

Physical changes that promote thrombosis include prolonged bed rest in the peripartum period and mechanical compression of the pelvic veins by the gravid uterus, leading to decreased venous return from the lower extremities, consecutive stasis, and the development of venous thrombosis [21].

2.8 Heparin-induced thrombocytopenia

Heparin-induced thrombocytopenia (HIT) is a condition mediated by the immune system through the development of heparin-dependent antibodies that have activated platelets, thereby increasing the risk of both venous and arterial thrombosis [15, 23].

IgG antibodies are directed against the antigenic complex formed by the binding of platelet factor 4 to heparin on the surface of platelets. This, in turn, activates surrounding platelets, leading to thrombin generation and the procoagulant state with the characteristic clinical manifestations of thrombocytopenia and thrombosis [23].

The diagnosis is confirmed by a decrease in platelets below 150,000/mL or by 50% from baseline in the presence of IgG HIT antibodies. The condition usually develops between 5 and 14 days after the start of heparin treatment, but may also develop within the first 24 hours in the case of previously administered heparin treatment. The risk is higher in surgical patients, especially following orthopedic and cardiac surgery, and is related to the period of exposure to heparin. Although heparin-induced thrombocytopenia is usually the result of treatment with unfractionated heparin, the occurrence of this condition has also been observed after administration of LMWH due to cross-reactivity between the two classes [15].

2.9 SARS-CoV-2

COVID-19 infection with severe acute respiratory syndrome coronavirus 2 has been shown to lead to a prothrombotic state, with variably reported incidences ranging from 11 to 70%, conditional on case severity and other predisposing factors.

The pathogen is thought to injure the vascular endothelium by attaching spike protein to the angiotensin-converting enzyme 2 receptors, thereby altering the properties of the endothelium into a thrombogenic surface, favoring platelet adhesion, hypercoagulability, and the development of micro or macrothrombosis at this level [11, 24].

3. Anticoagulation

Anticoagulant drugs are the first line of treatment for the prevention and treatment of thrombosis. This includes unfractionated heparin, low molecular weight heparin, fondaparinux, vitamin K antagonists (warfarin), and direct oral anticoagulants, which have a better safety profile than warfarin and have been shown to be equally effective, gradually replacing older agents [25].

The use of anticoagulants for primary prophylaxis has selected indications, such as for transient risk factors (prolonged hospitalization, postoperative status, certain orthopedic conditions) or may be considered for patients with high-risk hereditary thrombophilia, although for the latter there are not a large number of studies to support this indication [11, 26].

A patient who has developed a deep vein thrombosis and/or pulmonary embolism, whether provoked or unprovoked, should begin treatment with a direct oral anticoagulant for 3–6 months, according to the 2020 guidelines developed by the American Society of Hematology. It is also recommended that patients who have developed an unprovoked episode of deep vein thrombosis and/or pulmonary embolism or in whom a chronic risk factor can be identified should continue to receive secondary prophylaxis with either a standard or low-dose direct oral anticoagulant [10, 27].

For the purpose of secondary prophylaxis of various low-risk thrombophilias, the most recent studies recommend the use of direct oral anticoagulants instead of vitamin K antagonists, as the former possess a similar efficacy profile but with a better safety profile in terms of minor or major bleeding events. In high-risk thrombophilia, there is little data available to support the use of direct oral anticoagulants. A recent study testing the use of Rivaroxaban for secondary prophylaxis of high-risk antiphospholipid syndrome showed no additional benefit over traditional treatment, but an increased risk of bleeding [28, 29].

3.1 Factor V Leiden

In patients carrying the factor V Leiden mutation, no benefit of long-term anticoagulation has been shown in asymptomatic patients with no history of thrombosis. Although, short-term anticoagulation may be beneficial when other transient risk factors are identified. It is also recommended that women with or without a history of venous thromboembolism refrain from using estrogen-containing contraception and hormone replacement therapy [30].

Following an unprovoked venous thromboembolism event, the evidence favors long-term anticoagulation over short-term anticoagulation as secondary prophylaxis, although the duration has not been established but may be extended indefinitely if the risk of bleeding permits [31].

As a therapeutic agent, any direct oral anticoagulant can be used, as this is in line with the latest guidelines for the management of thromboembolism and the conclusion of several studies [29].

3.2 Prothrombin mutations

Carriers of heterozygous mutations, in the absence of other risk factors, do not require anticoagulation as primary prophylaxis [32].

After a first episode of deep vein thrombosis and/or pulmonary embolism associated with a reversible risk factor, it is recommended that the patient undergo anticoagulation therapy for at least 3 months, which may continue throughout life in case of recurrence [10, 32].

The initial treatment of venous thromboembolism is direct oral anticoagulation, although not all patient groups are suitable for this therapy, such as patients with antiphospholipid syndrome or extreme bodyweight. LMWH should be given before dabigatran and edoxaban [10, 32].

If treatment with direct oral anticoagulants is not possible, it is recommended to start warfarin therapy concomitantly with LMWH or fondaparinux for at least 5 days, monitoring INR, which should be in the range of 2.0–3.0 [33].

3.3 Factors C and S

The conclusion from the analysis of patients with factor C and S deficiency is limited by the lack of sufficient data to make specific recommendations, but it is safe to approach these patients from the point of view of venous thromboembolism management [10, 29].

Treatment of the first episode of venous thromboembolism should consist of unfractionated or LMWH for at least 5 days followed by vitamin k antagonists or DOAC for at least 3–6 months. In the presence of other clotting disorders or risk factors for thrombosis, or if the first episode was life-threatening or occurred in multiple sites, anticoagulation may be prolonged indefinitely [13].

3.4 Antiphospholipid syndrome

Primary prophylaxis with anticoagulant medication has not been shown to be beneficial for asymptomatic patients with no other risk factors, regardless of risk profile. Instead, some authors suggest daily administration of a low dose of aspirin, but this measure is not widely accepted. If other risk factors for thrombosis are associated, such as hospitalization, surgery, or concomitant autoimmune disease, prophylaxis is recommended, on a case-by-case basis [16, 34].

Secondary prophylaxis is recommended for patients with definite antiphospholipid syndrome and consists of lifelong vitamin K antagonist medication with a target INR of 2–3. In case of relapse or episodes of arterial thrombosis, the target INR should be >3. Combination with aspirin is not supported by data and is subject to controversy [16, 35].

The use of DOAC in patients with the definite antiphospholipid syndrome is not recommended, following the results of several studies that found direct oral anticoagulation to have a lower efficacy and safety profile than traditional vitamin K antagonist therapy [36].

3.5 Malignant conditions

Primary thromboprophylaxis of ambulatory cancer patients should be decided according to the individual risk of bleeding, the type of cancer, or the stage of the disease [37]. For hospitalized patients without acute venous thromboembolism or a history of venous thromboembolism, the American Society of Hematology recommends thromboprophylaxis with low molecular weight heparin, but only for the duration of the hospital stay. If during hospitalization a patient has undergone surgery or if a patient is receiving outpatient systemic chemotherapy and is at high risk of thrombosis, continued administration of LMWH has been shown to be beneficial. Oral anticoagulation, in the form of vitamin K antagonists or DOAC, is not included in current guidelines because there is insufficient data on its efficacy [38].

For a patient with active cancer who develops venous thromboembolism, initial treatment can be with either LMWH or DOAC, the latter being the medication of choice. It is recommended to continue treatment for at least 3–6 months, which may be extended as a secondary prophylactic measure in patients with active cancer and/or recurrence of venous thromboembolism. Direct oral anticoagulation remains the first choice of treatment in this case as well [38].

In a cancer patient with visceral or splanchnic venous thrombosis, according to the guidelines, treatment should consist of short-term anticoagulation (3–6 months) or clinical observation [38].

3.6 Pregnancy

Despite the prothrombotic status of physiological changes occurring during pregnancy, prophylactic anticoagulation of asymptomatic patients with no history of venous thromboembolism should be judged on a case-by-case basis [21, 39].

Anticoagulation for a venous thromboembolism event should be with LMWH if occurring before the 36th week of pregnancy and should be switched to unfractionated heparin afterward to minimize complications of epidural anesthesia. Vitamin K antagonists are not recommended after the first trimester as they are known to cause "warfarin embryopathy." Direct oral anticoagulation is also not approved for administration during pregnancy [21, 40].

Following an episode of venous thromboembolism, anticoagulation should be continued for 3–6 months, or 4–6 weeks postpartum, with either low molecular dose heparin or unfractionated heparin [21].

Patients with antiphospholipid syndrome and a history of thrombotic complications during previous pregnancies may benefit from prophylactic anticoagulation during pregnancy and for an additional 6 weeks postpartum [34].

3.7 SARS-CoV-2

Anticoagulation management of patients with Covid-19 depends on the severity of the disease. The administration of unfractionated heparin to patients hospitalized in an uncritical state has been observed to reduce the need for intensive care maneuvers, such as specific organ support or intubation, and also reduces the death rate. On the other hand, the condition of critically ill patients has not been improved by heparin treatment, and heparin treatment actually increases the rate of complications and is subsequently not recommended [41].

After discharge, patients with high thrombotic risk and a low bleeding risk could benefit from low-dose rivaroxaban treatment for an optimal duration to be determined [41].

4. Discussion/conclusion

A hypercoagulable state increases the patient's risk of developing arterial or venous thrombosis with subsequent complications. Venous thromboembolism is much more common, places a greater financial burden on health systems and therefore more data are available for its management.

Venous thromboembolism is now considered a multifaceted condition, usually resulting from the interaction of inherited and acquired risk factors, with different penetration in the general population and also with distinct risk profiles.

In terms of treatment, primary anticoagulant prophylaxis is recommended only for selected cases, while most patients require no treatment other than minimization of modifiable risk factors.

For the treatment of a first thrombotic event, secondary prophylaxis or relapse, anticoagulation is recommended. Although most episodes of a first thrombosis episode, especially when transient risk factors are identified, require short-term anticoagulation (3–6 months), there are cases where long-term (>6 months) or even indefinite anticoagulation may be given.

When choosing appropriate therapy, a large number of factors must be weighed, such as patient education, preference, and compliance for certain drugs, their availability for long-term follow-up, the financial burden of some therapies, or quality of life, for example when choosing between parenteral and oral treatment.

For patients with venous thromboembolism, the modern approved and guideline-supported treatment is DOAC, with superior efficacy and safety, and quality of life profiles compared to traditional vitamin K antagonist therapy. However, a limitation of DOAC is for the treatment of patients with high-risk antiphospholipid syndrome, where, in a recent study, DOAC showed no efficacy benefit but a higher risk compared to warfarin treatment.

Even though DOAC is finding an increasing number of indications, further research is needed to fully understand what is the best drug choice for each patient, for each condition, for the dose needed, for the duration of treatment, and for follow-up.

In conclusion, hypercoagulable conditions develop as a result of numerous individual or coexisting genetic or acquired risk factors that may be present and induce a higher risk for the patient to develop thrombotic complications. To prevent them, asymptomatic patients may have to undergo anticoagulant treatment in selected cases. For initial treatment and prevention of relapses, the modern and most recommended treatment is with direct anticoagulants, except for patients with high-risk antiphospholipid syndrome.

Author details

Iris Bararu Bojan, Stefan Dobreanu*, Oana Viola Badulescu, Maria Cristina Vladeanu, Andrei Bojan, Carmen Elena Plesoianu and Manuela Ciocoiu
Department of Internal Medicine, University of Medicine and Pharmacy "Grigore T. Popa" Iasi, Romania

*Address all correspondence to: stefan.dobreanu@yahoo.com

References

[1] Senst B, Tadi P, Goyal A, et al. Hypercoagulability. [Updated 2021 Sep 29]. In: StatPearls [Internet]. Treasure Island (FL): StatPearls Publishing; 2022 Jan-. Available from: https://www.ncbi.nlm.nih.gov/books/NBK538251/

[2] Kumar V, Abbas AK, Aster JC, Robbins SL. Hemostasis and Thrombosis. In: Robbins Basic Pathology. Essay. Philadelphia, PA: Elsevier/Saunders; 2013

[3] Alfirević Z, Alfirević I. Hypercoagulable state, pathophysiology, classification and epidemiology. Clinical Chemistry and Laboratory Medicine. Dec 2010;**48**(Suppl 1):S15-26. DOI: 10.1515/CCLM.2010.371. Epub 2010 Nov 16. PMID: 21077792

[4] Crowther MA. Congenital thrombophilic states associated with venous thrombosis: A qualitative overview and proposed classification system. Annals of Internal Medicine. 2003;**138**(2):128

[5] Stevens SM, Woller SC, Bauer KA, Kasthuri R, Cushman M, Streiff M, et al. Guidance for the evaluation and treatment of hereditary and acquired thrombophilia. Journal of Thrombosis and Thrombolysis. Jan 2016;**41**(1):154-164. DOI: 10.1007/s11239-015-1316-1. PMID: 26780744; PMCID: PMC4715840

[6] Thomas RH. Hypercoagulability syndromes. Archives of Internal Medicine. 2001;**161**(20):2433-2439. DOI: 10.1001/archinte.161.20.2433

[7] Albagoush SA, Koya S, Chakraborty RK, et al. Factor V Leiden Mutation. [Updated 2022 Feb 1]. In: StatPearls [Internet]. Treasure Island (FL): StatPearls Publishing; Jan 2022. Available from: https://www.ncbi.nlm.nih.gov/books/NBK534802/

[8] Kheradmand E, Haghjooy-Javanmard S, Dehghani L, Saadatnia M. Polymorphisms at activated protein C cleavage sites of factor V: Are they important in the absence of factor V Leiden?. Iranian Journal of Neurology. 2017;**16**(1):30-33

[9] Chan NC, Eikelboom JW, Weitz JI. Evolving Treatments for Arterial and Venous Thrombosis: Role of the Direct Oral Anticoagulants. Circulation Research. 29 Apr 2016;**118**(9):1409-1424. DOI: 10.1161/CIRCRESAHA.116.306925. PMID: 27126650

[10] Ortel TL, Neumann I, Ageno W, et al. American Society of Hematology 2020 guidelines for management of venous thromboembolism: Treatment of deep vein thrombosis and pulmonary embolism. Blood Advances. 2020;**4**(19):4693-4738. DOI: 10.1182/bloodadvances.2020001830

[11] Manojna Konda MD. Hereditary and Acquired Hypercoagulability. Practice Essentials, COVID-19, Pathophysiology. 2021

[12] Nicolaes GAF, Dahlbäck B. Congenital and acquired activated protein C resistance. Seminars in Vascular Medicine. Feb 2003;**3**(1):33-46. DOI: 10.1055/s-2003-38331. PMID: 15199491

[13] Gupta A, Tun AM, Gupta K, et al. Protein S Deficiency. [Updated 2021 Aug 29]. In: StatPearls [Internet]. Treasure Island (FL): StatPearls Publishing; Jan 2022. Available from: https://www.ncbi.nlm.nih.gov/books/NBK544344/

[14] Esmon CT. Protein S and protein C biochemistry, physiology, and clinical manifestation of deficiencies. Trends in Cardiovascular Medicine. 1992;**2**(6):214-219. DOI: 10.1016/1050-1738(92)90027-P

[15] Armstrong EM, Bellone JM, Hornsby LB, Treadway S, Phillippe HM. Acquired thrombophilia. Journal of Pharmacy Practice. 2014;**27**(3):234-242

[16] Tektonidou MG, Andreoli L, Limper M, et al. EULAR recommendations for the management of antiphospholipid syndrome in adults. Annals of the Rheumatic Diseases. 2019;**78**:1296-1304

[17] Abdol Razak NB, Jones G, Bhandari M, Berndt MC, Metharom P. Cancer-associated thrombosis: An overview of mechanisms, risk factors, and treatment. Cancers (Basel). 2018;**10**(10):380. Published 2018 Oct 11. DOI: 10.3390/cancers10100380

[18] Naess IA, Christiansen SC, Romundstad P, Cannegieter SC, Rosendaal FR, Hammerstrom J. Incidence and mortality of venous thrombosis: A population-based study. Journal of Thrombosis and Haemostasis: JTH. 2007;**5**(4):692-699

[19] Papageorgiou C, Jourdi G, Adjambri E, Walborn A, Patel P, Fareed J, et al. Disseminated intravascular coagulation: An update on pathogenesis, diagnosis, and therapeutic strategies. Clinical and Applied Thrombosis/Hemostasis: Official Journal of the International Academy of Clinical and Applied Thrombosis/Hemostasis. 2018;**24**(suppl. 9):8S-28S

[20] Tuzovic M, Herrmann J, Iliescu C, Marmagkiolis K, Ziaeian B, Yang EH. Arterial thrombosis in patients with cancer. Current Treatment Options in Cardiovascular Medicine. 2018;**20**(5):1-7

[21] Battinelli EM, Marshall A, Connors JM. The role of thrombophilia in pregnancy. Thrombosis. 2013;**2013**: 516420. DOI: 10.1155/2013/516420. Epub 2013 Dec 18. PMID: 24455235; PMCID: PMC3880751

[22] Bremme KA. Haemostatic changes in pregnancy. Best Practice & Research. Clinical Haematology. Jun 2003;**16**(2):153-168. DOI: 10.1016/s1521-6926(03)00021-5

[23] Linkins LA. Heparin induced thrombocytopenia. BMJ. 8 Jan 2015;**350**:g7566. DOI: 10.1136/bmj.g7566. PMID: 25569604

[24] Kichloo A, Dettloff K, Aljadah M, Albosta M, Jamal S, Singh J, et al. COVID-19 and hypercoagulability: A Review. Clinical and Applied Thrombosis Hemostasis. Jan-Dec 2020;**26**:1076029620962853. DOI: 10.1177/1076029620962853. PMID: 33074732; PMCID: PMC7592310

[25] Alquwaizani M, Buckley L, Adams C, Fanikos J. Anticoagulants: A review of the pharmacology, dosing, and complications. Current Emergency and Hospital Medicine Reports. 2013;**1**(2):83-97. Published 21 Apr 2013. DOI: 10.1007/s40138-013-0014-6

[26] Krumb E, Hermans C. Primary prophylaxis of venous thromboembolic disease with direct oral anticoagulants in patients with severe inherited thrombophilia. Research and Practice in Thrombosis and Haemostasis. 2021;**5**: 261-264. DOI: 10.1002/rth2.12479

[27] Donald Schreiber MD. Anticoagulation in Deep Venous Thrombosis: Advantages of Anticoagulant Therapy, Initial Anticoagulation Therapy, Long-Term Anticoagulation. 2021

[28] Campello E, Spiezia L, Simion C, Tormene D, Camporese G, Valle FD, et al. Direct oral anticoagulants in patients with inherited thrombophilia and venous thromboembolism: A prospective cohort study. Journal of the American Heart Association. 2020;**9**(23):e018917. DOI: 10.1161/JAHA.120.018917

[29] Elsebaie MAT, van Es N, Langston A, Büller HR, Gaddh M. Direct oral anticoagulants in patients with venous thromboembolism and thrombophilia: A systematic review and meta-analysis. Journal of Thrombosis and Haemostasis: JTH. 2019;**17**(4):645-656

[30] Kujovich JL. Factor V Leiden Thrombophilia. 14 May 1999 [Updated 2018 Jan 4]. In: Adam MP, Ardinger HH, Pagon RA, et al., editors. GeneReviews® [Internet]. Seattle (WA): University of Washington, Seattle; 1993-2022. Available from: https://www.ncbi.nlm.nih.gov/books/NBK1368/

[31] Donovan AK, Smith KJ, Ragni MV. Anticoagulation duration in heterozygous factor V Leiden: a decision analysis. Thrombosis Research. 2013;**132**(6):724-728. DOI: 10.1016/j.thromres.2013.09.012. [Epub Sep 16 2013]. PMID: 24112753.

[32] Kujovich JL. Prothrombin Thrombophilia. 2006 Jul 25 [Updated 2021 Feb 4]. In: Adam MP, Ardinger HH, Pagon RA, et al., editors. GeneReviews® [Internet]. Seattle (WA): University of Washington, Seattle; 1993-2022. Available from: https://www.ncbi.nlm.nih.gov/books/NBK1148/

[33] Bani-Hani S, Siddiqui O, Patel A, Showkat A. C20209T prothrombin gene mutation associated deep venous thrombosis in a hemodialysis Patient. Clinical Nephrology. Case Studies. 2014;**2**:1-4. Published 2014 Jan 15. DOI: 10.5414/CNCS107984

[34] Suneel Movva MD. Antiphospholipid Syndrome Treatment & Management: Medical care, surgical care, consultations. Antiphospholipid Syndrome Treatment & Management: Medical Care, Surgical Care, Consultations. 2021

[35] Del Papa N, Vaso N. Management of antiphospholipid syndrome. Therapeutic Advances in Musculoskeletal Disease. 2010;**2**(4):221-227. DOI: 10.1177/1759720X10365969

[36] Dufrost V, Risse J, Zuily S, Wahl D. Direct oral anticoagulants use in antiphospholipid syndrome: Are these drugs an effective and safe alternative to Warfarin? A systematic review of the literature. Current Rheumatology Reports. 2016;**18**(12):74. DOI: 10.1007/s11926-016-0623-7

[37] Park J, Lee JM, Lee JS, Cho YJ. Pharmacological and mechanical thromboprophylaxis in critically ill patients: A network meta-analysis of 12 trials. Journal of Korean Medical Science. 2016;**31**(11):1828-1837. DOI: 10.3346/jkms.2016.31.11.1828

[38] Lyman GH, Carrier M, Ay C, Di Nisio M, Hicks LK, Khorana AA, et al. American Society of Hematology 2021 guidelines for management of venous thromboembolism: Prevention and treatment in patients with cancer. Blood Advances. 23 Feb 2021;**5**(4):927-974. DOI: 10.1182/bloodadvances.2020003442. Erratum in: Blood Adv. 2021 Apr 13;5(7):1953. PMID: 33570602; PMCID: PMC7903232

[39] Dargaud Y, Rugeri L, Vergnes MC, Arnuti B, Miranda P, Negrier C, et al. A risk score for the management of pregnant women with increased risk of

venous thromboembolism: A multicentre prospective study. British Journal of Haematology. 2009;**145**(6):825-835

[40] Regitz-Zagrosek V, Roos-Hesselink JW, Bauersachs J, Blomström-Lundqvist C, Cífková R, De Bonis M, et al. 2018 ESC Guidelines for the Management of Cardiovascular Diseases during Pregnancy: The Task Force for the Management of Cardiovascular Diseases during Pregnancy of the European Society of Cardiology (ESC). European Heart Journal. September 2018;**39**(34), 07:3165-3241. DOI: 10.1093/eurheartj/ehy340

[41] Lopes RD, de Barros E, Silva P, Furtado R, Macedo A, Bronhara B, et al. Therapeutic versus prophylactic anticoagulation for patients admitted to hospital with COVID-19 and elevated D-dimer concentration (ACTION): An open-label, multicentre, randomised, controlled trial. Lancet (London, England). 2021;**397**(10291):2253-2263

Section 2

Individual Disease Conditions

Chapter 3

Use of Non-Vitamin K-Dependent Oral Anticoagulants in Elderly and Fragile Patients with Atrial Fibrillation

Ortigoza Daniel Víctor

Abstract

Atrial fibrillation is a frequently observed entity in medical practice, with cases on the rise if we focus on age groups of frail elderly patients. It is important to identify them since advanced age and comorbidities suppose greater numbers of cases of thromboembolic diseases and strokes, entities that can be prevented with the non-vitamin K antagonist oral anticoagulants (NOACs), managing a balance between prevention and safety and thus avoiding complications, for this, a correct search and screening must be made to reach the largest number of patients who could benefit from this therapy. Old age is not a synonym of frailty, so, we must be cautious with the loss of autonomy of our patients and we must have a multidisciplinary approach to accompany this increasingly frequent and extended period, being very alert to drug interactions and decreased daily life skills.

Keywords: elderly, direct oral anticoagulants, fragility, nonagenarian, non-vitamin K antagonist oral anticoagulants, atrial fibrillation, anticoagulation

1. Introduction

Atrial fibrillation (AF) is the most common supraventricular arrhythmia in the elderly in daily medical practice, with a correlation of decade-by-decade growth in the world population, being the onset and may also be part of various concomitant diseases that worsen the health of the population.

In the elderly patient, AF anticoagulation is used to prevent systemic embolic events (SEE) and stroke phenomena and their consequences; vascular dementia; worsening of heart failure (HF) and kidney function, among other pathologies.

In the indication of anticoagulation, the use of direct oral anticoagulants (DOACs) is gaining ground over treatment with vitamin K antagonist (VKA), this is due to their easy use of the indicated medication, their wide therapeutic window, the few adverse effects, and extensive support of scientific information that supports them.

The four large randomized pivotal works in Non-Valvular Atrial Fibrillation (NVAF) on anticoagulation [1–4] have included approximately 27,000 patients, mostly under 75 years of age, so later works were generated with observational evidence from the database in different countries on patients over 75 years of age, octogenarians and, a little less, in nonagenarians and patients over 90 years old.

Frailty has taken on a notorious relevance in recent decades due to the increase in life expectancy, thanks to improvements in the care of elderly patients, better medical treatments, and early diagnoses of comorbidities.

The age segment of nonagenarians has constant growth worldwide, and in addition, this group of patients, who suffer greater comorbidities and increase in embolic episodes, which can be prevented, gives rise to a dilemma that we hope to clarify, the fears of anticoagulation and the benefits of using DOACs.

2. An elderly patient with AF

2.1 Epidemiology

The elderly world population >65 years old in 2004 was 461 million, and it is estimated that it will grow 4.3 times by 2050 [5].

The challenge proposed by diagnosing a supraventricular arrhythmia, as frequent as atrial fibrillation (AF), is important to avoid future complications, such as systemic embolism (SEE) diseases, stroke, heart failure, tachycardiomyopathies, worsening cognitive disorders and dementia, increased fragility syndrome, and polypharmacy.

AF screening in the elderly population is of paramount importance. It is at 4.6% which positions it in a perfect cost-benefit balance (it takes only 70 elderly individuals to find a patient with AF) [6].

2.2 Diagnosis of AF in the elderly

AF can be detected in the patient in different medical areas, such as in an emergency service, in clinical consultation, in a pre-competitive check-up for sports, and in an immediate postoperative period.

Semiology should be used with the simple manual pulse socket or with different devices; electrical tensiometers, smartwatches, and in those who have some type of external monitoring the multi parameters, Holter, etc., or some instrument for internal monitoring are the loop recover, pacemakers, defibrillators, etc. In this way, it is about looking for, when interrogating these devices, the atrial high-frequency episodes (AHFE) characteristic of AF, which will then be corroborated with 12-lead electrocardiogram "Gold Standard" to be able to make the diagnosis of clinical AF and if it cannot be compared with ECG, it will be a subclinical AF.

In elderly patients, it is recommended to use the nominal classification of AF; previously undiagnosed AF, paroxysmal AF, persistent AF, long-term persistent AF, and permanent AF. All AF modalities must be anticoagulated or look for all the tools to be able to do so, except those that are contraindicated [6].

One term that falls into disuse is Non-Valvular Atrial Fibrillation (NVAF) [6, 7] which encompasses all AF except those for which anticoagulation with DOACs does not represent a benefit; moderate or severe mitral stenosis and those concomitant with mechanical heart valves.

In an elderly patient with NVAF, the thromboembolic probability he/she suffers must be weighted, by using the CHA_2DS_2VASc scale [8] where it is established that the elderly patient who is ≥75 years old, provides information to establish a crucial score of 2, with an embolic probability of 4% per year, and if the patient is also female, 1 point with this sum of data, anticoagulation is a priority (Class I A) [9].

When the stroke prevention score is established, the probability of bleeding should be assessed with the HAS-BLED scale, which is a daily example of a 65-year-old patient with knee osteoarthritis, added to this a history of the previous stroke, who drinks wine daily and the use of nonsteroidal anti-inflammatory drugs (NSAIDs), gives a count of four with a probability of bleeding of 4.9–1.9% annually. But it is advisable to suppress alcohol consumption and change the type of painkillers to non-NSAIDs, the eventuality of future bleeding is reduced to 1.88–3.2% per year [10].

Glomerular Filtration Rate (GFR) is another important factor to be able to assess renal function with a calculation formula, "Crockoft Goul formula" (CG) estimated by the patient's serum creatinine, age, weight, and a constant numeric denominator. The result of this equation is corrected in the case of female patients [9, 11].

When studying healthy elderly people aged 70–101 years, a significant correlation between age and GFR measured with CG was observed, where it was concluded that GFR figures decrease by 1.01 ml/min per year [12].

An anticoagulation card was designed to be taken to each medical consultation and which includes useful tools to help decide on anticoagulation and to make dose corrections at each medical visit if the patient required it (**Figure 1**).

Once it is decided to treat with anticoagulant an elderly patient, the challenge is to choose the right anticoagulant for each patient. DOACs or Warfarin? If you choose the first one, the options are—dabigatran, rivaroxaban, apixaban, or edoxaban. An attempt will be made to bring the right option closer during this chapter.

2.3 Elderly anticoagulated patient

In the pivotal trials on anticoagulation in patients with NVAF, individuals with an average age of 70 years, small ethnic groups, with a lower percentage of women, and none with renal failure on dialysis enrolled.

The four large studies, such as ARISTOTLE included 3658 patients >75 (31%); in RE-LAY, n = 7258 (40%); in a subgroup of ROCKET-AF, N = 6259 (44%) and in the ENGAGE AF-TIMI 48 trial, n = 8474, (40.05%).

All this forceful but scarce information in relation to the elderly led to multiple analyses of real-life data.

In 2017, a group of patients (n = 110) who were between 66 and 100 years old (average age of 80.4 years) was studied, of which 45% were women. The use of apixaban at maximum doses of 5 mg every 12 hours or doses lower than 2.5 every 12 hours was observed when they met 2 of 3 criteria stipulated in the ARISTOTLE study (>80 years, weight < 60 kg, and plasma creatinine >1.5 mg/dl).

Patients who received the maximum recommended doses, approximately 10% had drug concentrations above the expected range, as did 2/3 of the patients who used apixaban 2.5 mg every 12 hours.

Differences in the proportion of apixaban concentrations within or outside the expected ranges were not significantly different. However, four patients had apixaban dosage above the expected range.

This increase in drug concentrations found in this small group of elderly people could allow the possibility of a blood dosage of the anticoagulant drug, to minimize inconveniences, since these patients, old as such, have not been taken into account in large randomized studies [13].

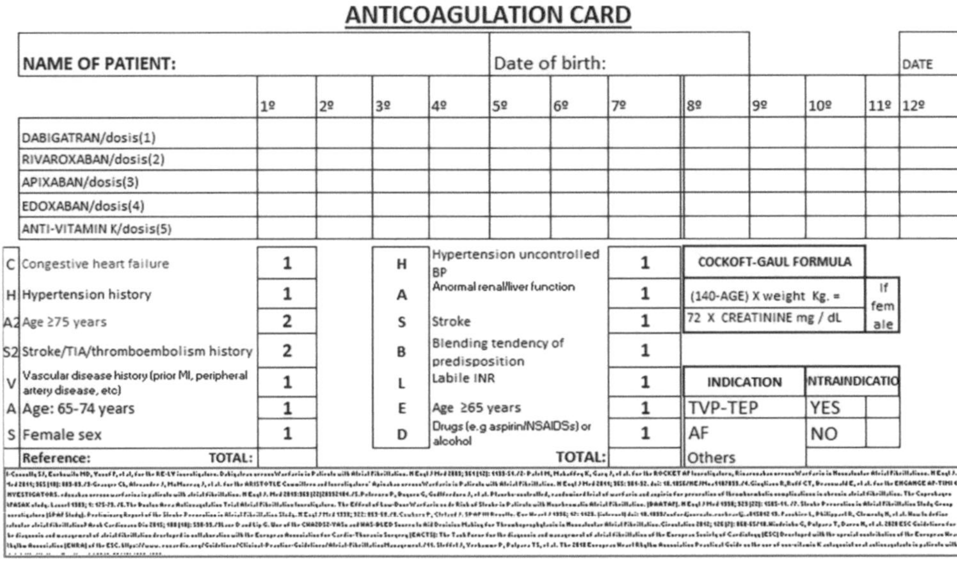

ANTICOAGULATION CARD

NAME OF PATIENT:					Date of birth:							DATE
	1º	2º	3º	4º	5º	6º	7º	8º	9º	10º	11º	12º
DABIGATRAN/dosis(1)												
RIVAROXABAN/dosis(2)												
APIXABAN/dosis(3)												
EDOXABAN/dosis(4)												
ANTI-VITAMIN K/dosis(5)												

C	Congestive heart failure	1	H	Hypertension uncontrolled BP	1
H	Hypertension history	1	A	Anormal renal/liver function	1
A2	Age ≥75 years	2	S	Stroke	1
S2	Stroke/TIA/thromboembolism history	2	B	Blending tendency of predisposition	1
V	Vascular disease history (prior MI, peripheral artery disease, etc)	1	L	Labile INR	1
A	Age: 65-74 years	1	E	Age ≥65 years	1
S	Female sex	1	D	Drugs (e.g aspirin/NSAIDSs) or alcohol	1
	Reference: TOTAL:			TOTAL:	

COCKOFT-GAUL FORMULA

(140-AGE) X weight Kg. = / 72 X CREATININE mg / dL — If female

INDICATION	NTRAINDICATIO
TVP-TEP	YES
AF	NO
Others	

Figure 1.
Anticoagulation card. Anticoagulation card to be used by the patient at each medical visit.

In a Canadian meta-analysis of three cohorts (n = 227,579) in which different DOACs were compared (rivaroxaban vs. dabigatran, apixaban vs. dabigatran, and apixaban vs. rivaroxaban). It served to assess each other's effectiveness and safety.

The follow-up period was approximately 5 years, with an average participation age close to 75 years, with a low percentage of women, CHA2SD2VASC = 2.5. These patients were treated with high doses and reduced doses of non-vitamin K antagonist oral anticoagulants (NOACs).

The meta-analysis concludes that apixaban in these elderly patients was associated with fewer ischemic stroke events and systemic embolic (ES). When compared to rivaroxaban, a 15% decrease was found, and with respect to major bleeding (MB) the data obtained in favor of apixaban was 39% [14].

Regarding dabigatran in the RE-LAY study compared to warfarin when segmented by age in over 75 years of age (n = 7258), it significantly reduced stroke and intracerebral hemorrhage (ICH) and was also shown that at a dose of 110 mg every 12 hours it is a safe option for patients >80 years old when it comes to reducing the slight increase in extracranial bleeding [15].

Based on the ROCKET-AF study, where 44% of patients were >75 years old, rivaroxaban prevented stroke and reduced bleeding in life-threatening critical anatomical areas and bleeding from all causes. The reduction of the hemorrhagic stroke was 41%, with a $p < 0.02$). This group of patients was more polymorphic and they benefit from the use of rivaroxaban if they had the previous stroke as history, both young and elderly patients [16].

In 2015, 30,655 patients >75 years old were recruited in eight studies published as a meta-analysis. The different DOACs vs. warfarin (two studies for apixaban, n = 2850; one study for dabigatran, n = 2466; two studies for edoxaban, n = 2838; three studies for rivaroxaban, n = 3082) were compared with a follow-up of 3 months to 2.8 years.

This meta-analysis evaluated the efficacy of each drug in elderly people with stroke events and systemic embolisms (ES), also MB and clinically nonrelevant mayor bleeding (CNRMB).

All DOACs compared to warfarin were significantly better, by an average of 29%. Regarding safety, edoxaban and apixaban turned out to be more beneficial in this group of elderly. Dabigatran in doses of 150 mg and 110 mg, both in two daily doses, had a higher number of gastrointestinal (GI) bleeding, along with rivaroxaban, which also had a lower safety profile (**Figures 2** and **3**) [17].

Based on data collected in the Norwegian patient registry and the database of the same country, from 2012 to 2017, where the use of NOACs (standard dose and reduced doses) vs. warfarin is compared, it was observed.

The total population studied was 31,041 of >75 years (average 82 years), 52% women with an average of $CHA_2DS_2VASC = 4.5$.

The use of DOACs in standard and reduced doses decreased stroke and systemic embolism like warfarin, but the administration of low doses of DOACs is either similar or reduces bleeding complications. A door could be opened for future randomized subdose studies [18].

Three prespecified groups of edoxaban vs. warfarin were studied, with a follow-up of approximately 2.8 years, in patients with NVAF. The third group, >75 years old, had 52% permanent AF. The direct oral factor Xa inhibitor was used in the standard and reduced doses, the latter by 41%.

About 2.3% stroke and SEE were observed, 4.8% of MB with significant data. Embolisms were reduced by 17% and the same percentage of reduction was achieved in bleeding, so a safety tool is provided in the elderly when compared to younger patient groups [19].

START T Register 2, studied in people over 85 years of age, showed that using DOACs there was low mortality, similar bleeding when compared to warfarin treatment. In addition, a small increase was observed in very elderly patients with embolic events with the use of direct oral anticoagulants [20].

The use of warfarin has its disadvantages in long-lived patients; such as the need for frequent measurements of the International Normalized Ratio (INR), which is not always in a standardized window, and therefore has the difficulty in entering the Time in Therapeutic Range (TTR).

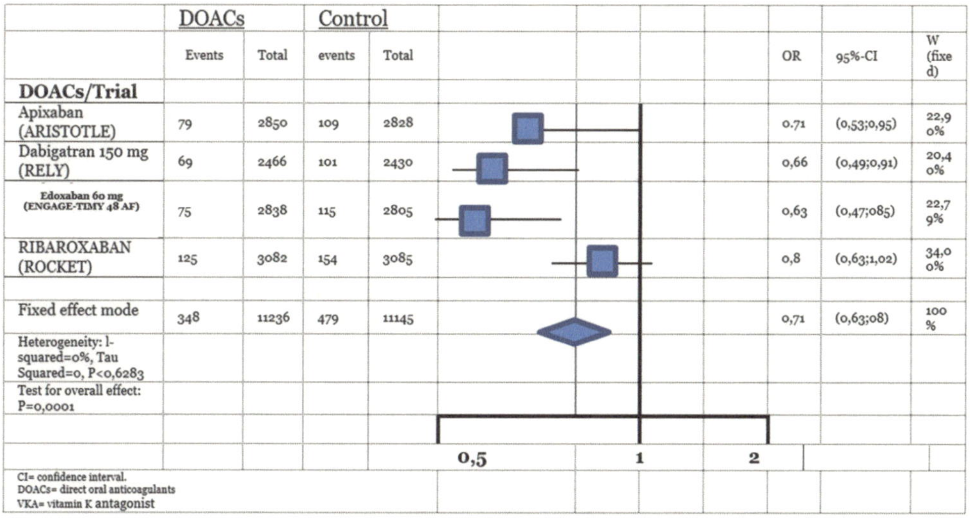

Figure 2.
Stroke and systemic embolism in subjects older than 75 years with DOACs.

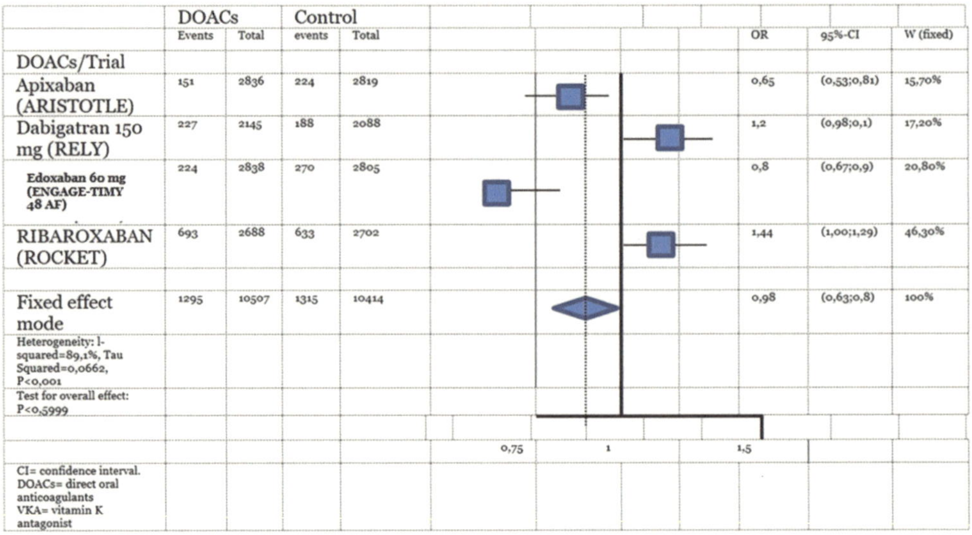

Figure 3.
Major bleeding and clinically nonrelevant bleeding in patients over 75 years of age with DOACs.

Warfarin interrupts the necessary recycling of vitamin K, which is an essential cofactor for the carboxylation of glutamic residues responsible for producing proteins indispensable for clotting. An example of this is the decrease in protein C levels, which can favor calcium deposits in the skin and other organs; as well as, this vitamin is required in the primary phases of bone matrix formation, effects of paramount importance in this advanced age group [21, 22].

In a database, a retrospective cohort of the city of Taiwan was observed (n = 17,008), an average of 28% reduction in osteoporosis was observed when comparing DOACs vs. warfarin.

DOACs, especially the use of apixaban, minimize osteoporosis by 62% and rivaroxaban also does so by 32%, a decrease that is not statistically significant in those compared to dabigatran [23].

DOACs do not deteriorate the γ-carboxylation of osteoclastine and do not disfavor the formation of the bone matrix, a very interesting topic for good "bone health."

3. Frail patient with AF

3.1 Epidemiology

The collection of information and quantification on fragility syndrome leads to analyzing a wide range of data dispersion, from different ethnic groups, various forms of measurements, in addition to the disparate life expectancy in different countries.

Fragility in the US has a higher incidence in white ethnicity [24], in Latin America and the Caribbean, there is data of great percentage disintegration, from 7.7 to 42%, with an average of 19.6% (data surpassed in North America, Europe, and Oceania) [25].

Atrial fibrillation (AF) is the unprevalent supraventricular arrhythmia in the young population, 2–3 cases per 1000 inhabitants, but the number of cases grows considerably to 50–90 per 1000 people ranging from 62 to 92 years [26, 27], and its number will multiply by 2.5 times by 2050 [9, 28], the product of its greater emphasis on the detection of arrhythmia.

The finding can range from the simple taking of the pulse looking for its classic irregularity to the need to search for information through the use of implanted devices (pacemaker, cardio-defibrillators, loop recorder) or diagnostic methods, such as 24-hour Holter, smartwatches, pulse meters.

In fragile patients, AF is more frequent, although the data can widely vary from 4.4–75% by different measurement modalities [29].

In a systematic review that included 21 studies, from 1998 to 2010 on four continents, with a total of 61,500 participants over 65 years of age, a variable range of data ranging from 4.0% to 59.1% was found with a fragility prevalence of 10.7% (95% CI = 10.5–10.9). As is already known, this percentage increases with age and female sex with significant statistical data of $p < 0.001$; and when talking about pre-fragility, the percentage found is close to 42% [30].

The Framingham Heart Study shows us that age as a solitary variable is sufficient predictive value in elderly people aged 80–90 years to increase the probability of suffering a stroke or transient ischemic attack (stroke/TIA) by 23.5%. In this population follow-up, one in three people of European descent will suffer from AF throughout their lives [31, 32].

In the totality of patients over 85 years of age, between a quarter and half of the patients are fragile, so it could be considered, who expect that two-thirds of the long-lived population could be prevented or detected to avoid disabilities.

3.2 Definition

Fragility as a syndrome is more frequent in patients in the last decades of their lives. It is characterized by a state of greater vulnerability, where different stressors contribute to the loss of physiological reserves, with the subsequent rupture of the homeostatic balance.

The most frequent stressors that trigger this physiological harmony can be of different characteristics; from chronic conditions, such as diabetes mellitus, chronic obstructive disease, skin infections, such as erysipelas, respiratory sequelae left by COVID-19, heart failure, atrial fibrillation, hip fracture, and long periods of bed rest, stroke, loss of loved ones, widowhood, loneliness, and low economic level.

Fried et al. in 2004 [33] establishes a clinical syndrome, describing the presence of three or more criteria that are summarized in **Figure 4**.

When the loss of physiological reserves is affected by two noxas, it is called pre-fragility, which when new noxas are added to them, becomes fragility syndrome. Subsequently, if more decompensating factors are added, a dreaded disability could arise (**Figure 5**) [34].

3.3 Fragile patient assessment tools

To recognize fragility early, a comprehensive assessment is needed, using clinical, functional, behavioral and biological markers [35, 36] that can help measure or quantify through the weighting Activity of Daily Living (ADLs), using the Katz index (eating, clothing, personal hygiene, bathroom use, continence management, and mobility). At earlier stages, you can use the assessment of the Instrumental Activity

Clinical critters	Score
Weight loss More than 5kg or 5% of the total corporal weight, on a year	1
Self-reported exhaustion Lower than 20% pressuring strength of normality by BMI	1
Low energy expenditure Weariness	1
Slow gait speed More than 20% of normality index limit stratified by sex and height to walk 4.57 m	1
Low percent of physical activity/ calculation of adjusted daily calorie consume	1

BMI (body index mass)

Figure 4.
Clinical characteristics of fragility.

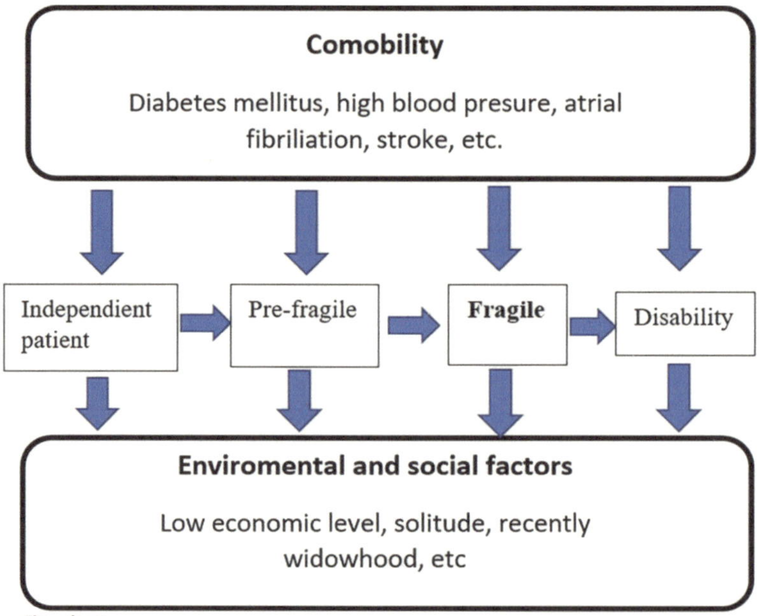

Flowchart

Figure 5.
Progressive deteriorate of independent patient.

of Daily Living (IADLs), measured by the LOWTON index (use of the phone, shopping, preparing meals, take care of your home, laundry, use of transport, the correct taking of your own medication, the management of the home economy) [37] and the Charlson comorbidity index [38, 39].

If the evolution of the clinical phenotype of fragility is followed at 3 years, F patients with lower economic resources suffer greater comorbidities, such as frequent falls, stroke, thus worsening mobility and ADLs [40].

3.4 Fragility and anticoagulation

The interest in information on anticoagulation and fragility is growing, thanks to more available information and a better understanding on the subject that being elderly is not the same as having fragility syndrome. Although many elderly individuals suffer from three frequent criteria, such as physical fatigue, weight loss, and slowness when traveling, these items can be reversed if patients are educated in better nutrition, regulated weekly physical activity, if possible with the supervision of trained staff (aquagym, hiking, Tai Chi, etc.) and in turn prevent sarcopenia with improvements in postural balancing and in this way, falls would be avoided [41].

Age ≥ 75 years provides the crucial points to prevent the probabilities of thromboembolism (TE) and stroke with anticoagulants (OACs), according to the CHA_2DS_2VASCS score in patients with NVAF.

This data is relevant, since, for example, it was observed in 2018, in Argentina, it had registered 31,700 visits per year to a Hospital Emergency Service with a large dispersion in the age range, the average age of 75 years was recorded [42].

Fumagalli et al. studied frail elderly patients older than 70 years with AF (10%) in 14 European countries; they were divided into three age groups. It was observed that 37% of patients, medicated with DOAC (37%) and 5.7% of individuals who cannot be given anticoagulants, were treated with left atrial appendage closure (LAAC).

Less than 11% of the treating physicians considered age as an individual factor for not medicating with anticoagulants, a fact not sufficiently explained by the authors [43].

In a survey conducted in 41 European centers, patients considered fragile and their influence on the management of arrhythmia was studied. AF was found in 72% of patients.

About 57% were diagnosed as fragile patients; 29% were pre-fragile; and 8% of the studied population was >85 years old, which had a higher number of comorbidities and higher rate of drug use, data that reached statistical significance [44].

In relation to falls and the use of DOACs, two studies were carried out; the first was a retrospective subanalysis of ARISTOTLE. It included 753 patients aged 65–74 years, who suffered falls and had a greater number of comorbidities. An 80% benefit was observed in terms of the reduction of intracerebral hemorrhage (ICH) when compared to this group of patients, the use of apixaban vs. that of warfarin [45].

In the second prospective study, a subanalysis of ENGANGE AF, TIMI 48 where patients were treated with edoxaban or warfarin, patients who had falls and those who did not have it were analyzed.

This observed population group (n = 900), older (average 77 years), with more comorbidities (Charlson Comorbidities Index > 5, CHA_2DS_2VASC > 5, HAS-BLED > 3, 50% permanent AF), had a reduction in mortality and significant severe bleeding, with a considerable decrease in the dreaded intracerebral hemorrhage (ICH) [46].

In the analysis of a subgroup of ARISTOPHANES, considered the largest retrospective observational study using a US database, from 2013 to 2015, they were a population group of fragile elderly people with NVAF with an average age of 83–84 years. Comparing cohorts of patients medicated with DOACS (apixaban, dabigatran, and rivaroxaban) or warfarin, significant weights were established referring to stroke/ES and MB risks [47].

All patients with AF were 150,487, 34% of these were fragile, 90% had a CHA_2DS_2VASc score ≥ 4, taken as a high risk of stroke, and in more than 80% a HAS-BLED ≥ 3, was considered a threat to bleeding.

Better response with respect to SEE and stroke risk was found with patients who received apixaban (49%) and rivaroxaban (21%), compared to those treated with warfarin.

In relation to MB, apixaban (38%) and dabigatran (21%) had less bleeding and with regard to rivaroxaban vs. warfarin, in the former, there was a small increase in bleeding.

In the SAFIR Cohort study, 995 fragile elderly people were admitted to 33 centers and then followed for a year, it was sought to compare the use of rivaroxaban vs. warfarin.

This group of elderly people with many comorbidities was made up of 23% of nonagenarian people, almost half suffered from a decrease in kidney function, 77% high blood pressure, 50% malnourished, 41% anemia, 39% dementia, and 27% falls (an average of the different scores: CHA_2DS_2VASc = 4.8, HAS-BLED = 2.3, mini-mental test = 21.5, activities of daily life 4.4, CCI = 6.7).

When comparing the two Cohorts (rivaroxaban vs. warfarin), adjusted to comorbidities, age, and previous treatment, fragile elderly patients who used rivaroxaban had a significant reduction in MB of 33%, a lower percentage of ICH of 48%, with no differences in mortality decrease and stroke [48].

So, the use of DOACs in fragile patients is a good therapeutic alternative, due to the wide use in the treatment of these patients, wide therapeutic range, predictable pharmacokinetics, easy administration, and little drug interaction; without the need for frequent monitoring and dose adjustment, what is very important in this age group.

The fragile patient is significantly vulnerable due to the polypharmacy by which the use of DOACs in AF dispenses with therapeutic bridge with low molecular weight heparin and helps expand the range of a better diet, being able to incorporate leafy vegetables, contained with the use of vitamin K antagonist [49].

4. Nonagenarian patient with AF

4.1 Epidemiology

Improvements in health systems and education in human care progressively lead to an increase in life expectancy, especially in developed countries.

The population census of Spain 2021 had a total of 47,394,223 inhabitants, with a record of 491,369 (1.03%) individuals ≥90 years old [50]. In Argentina, 45,808,747 people were projected for 2021, of whom 242,409 (0.53%) would be ultra-elderly people [51].

In Germany, according to population growth projection data in 2021, the total population of 83,450,000 and is expected by 2030 to be 82,857,000, with a slight population decrease of 593,000 people (0.71%). Paradoxically, the numerical count of residents will increase in the age group ≥90 years, from 878,000 to 1.40,300 (1.69%); and in this way, it is speculated that the number of very long-lived individuals will grow by 59.79% [52].

In the prospective longitudinal study in Gothenburg, Sweden, which initiated the enrolment of patients at 70 years and was then followed for 30 years; an AF prevalence of 16.8% at 90 years was recorded, with an incidence of approximately 47/1000/year in both sexes; and in the 95–99-year group (n = 189) it had an almost double incidence of 93/1000/year; with an increase in men [53].

4.2 Anticoagulated nonagenarian patient

In the subanalysis of very elderly patients with NVAF, J-RHYTHM registry, 7406 consecutive individuals were enrolled who were divided into three age groups (<70 years; 70–84 years, and >85 years).

This elderly population of the third age group with the highest preponderance to polypathologies (n = 330) had an average age of 87.4 ± 2.8 (4.4%), with 58.8% permanent AF. The combination of thrombus embolism and major bleeding was lower in those who used warfarin at an International Normalized Ratio (INR) between 1.6 and 2.59 with a $p < 0.001$.

The registry compared the ultra-elders the use of warfarin with a TTR of 67.1 vs. the other group, those who did not use warfarin. It was postulated that it could be used in very long-lived, with a lower INR range than that used in large anticoagulation works [54].

Based on the National Registry of Taiwan 2012, T.-F. Chao et al. [55] investigated patients >90 years with NVAF in a total of n = 16,798 with an average age of 92.5 years.

N = 7362 were observed with different pre-existing diseases, such as chronic kidney disease, n = 3151 (CKD); intracerebral bleeding, n = 950 (ICH); and gastrointestinal bleeding, n = 5370 (GI).

About 67.3% of the patients studied, n = 4955, were not treated with anticoagulants (N-OACs), and 32.7%, n = 2407 were anticoagulated (OACs).

Of the OAC, DOACs was used in 23.6%; apixaban (n = 190), 2.6%; rivaroxaban (n = 927), 12.6%; dabigatran (n = 620), 8.4%; as a vitamin K antagonist, warfarin (n = 670), 9.1%.

Rivaroxaban was the most used DOACs in doses of 10 mg, 15 mg, and 20 mg once a day, with a preference of treating physicians with doses of rivaroxaban 15 mg/day at 41%. Regarding apixaban, the doses of 2.5 mg every 12 hours and dabigatran 110 mg twice a day were the most frequently chosen drug presentations (**Figure 6**) [55].

A total of 1750 patients with AF >90 years of age were identified from three regions of Spain, these enrolled individuals were divided into three groups; the nonanticoagulated n = 534; those anticoagulated with vitamin K antagonist (VKA), n = 500 with INR = 2–3. Those who were treated with DOACs, n = 716. Patients had a creatinine clearance close to 50 ml/min [56].

In a subanalysis of the FREFER-AF study, 6412 adult patients with AF were enrolled and followed for 12 months. In this European registry, they were divided into three age groups (<85 years old; >85 years old; and >90 years old), 505 patients were very old >85 years old and referred to the third group (16.6%), 84 of them were extremely elderly.

This segment of ultra-elderly people suffered a net clinical benefit when they were anticoagulated with DOACs, a balance given by a reduction in thromboembolic events of 43%, which is evident when treating 50 individuals to avoid an event.

A significant difference was established in favor of anticoagulantes of 4.6%; $p < 0.48$, with an increase in major bleeding similar to patients >75 years (younger), the comparison was made by age groups who took only anticoagulants, only anti-platelets, or the sum of the two, $p < 0.025$.

Regarding MB, it had only a 10% increase compared to the extremely elderly (>90) who were not anticoagulated.

The net clinical benefit is observed in the three groups, with greater intensity in those over 90 years of age, being 8.02% with a $p < 0036$ (**Figure 7**) [57].

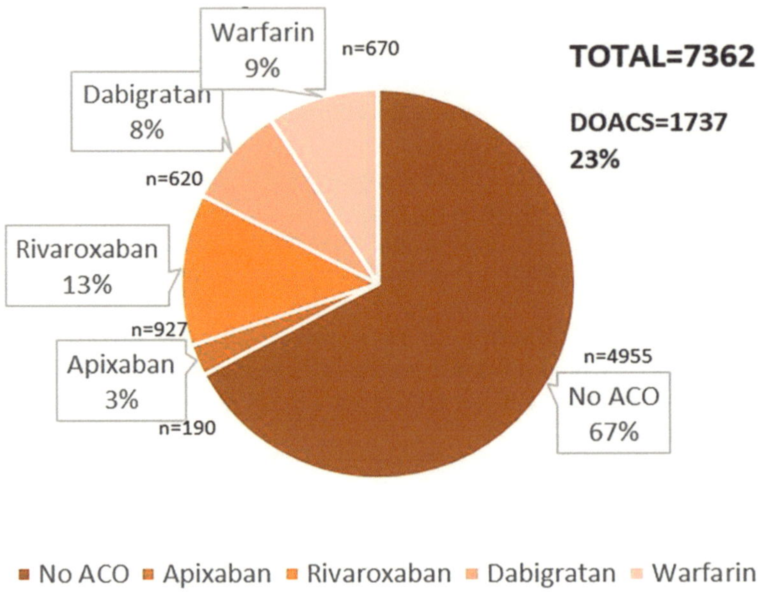

Figure 6.
Patients >90 with AF and history of previous illnesses.

It was found among the best net benefit of reducing embolic phenomena and bleeding to anticoagulated patients >90 years old (6.1% use of DOACs).

Nonagenarian patients aged 90–100.1 years (n = 300) with an age average of 91 years who suffered from AF and were medicated with OACs were studied.

Extremely elderly individuals were divided into three groups; those who took DOACs (n = 93), those who took warfarin (n = 147), and a third group (N-OACs) n = 80 who were not medicated with anticoagulants.

Regarding the stroke/TIA/SEE the DOACs were statistically significant reduction (**Figure 8**) and it was observed on the bleeding events the DOACs had twice the percentage of bleeding—5%/year vs. 2.5% from warfarin use (p < 0.048) (**Figure 9**) [58].

As already observed, in the subanalysis of the START-T Register, done in Italy, patients enrolled from 2012 to 2013, elderly people with NVAF, who were mostly treated with warfarin as an anticoagulant since the spread of the use of DOACs was beginning in this country. Two-thirds of the elderly were observed to have moderate or severe kidney disease [20].

In the START-T Registry 2 subanalysis, elderly people enrolled with VNAF, with average age 88.4 ± 2.8, compared DOACs (41.3%) vs. warfarin in the range 2–3 (58.7%).

The study was divided into two groups, <85 years and >85 years (n = 3209), in the second group, >90 years out of age 55 patients (1.7%).

In very elderly patients it was obtained; a mortality rate and a lower risk of sacred with a small thromboembolic increase [59].

In the Swedish design of 30 years of follow-up of patients with and without AF, separated by sex, it was observed that among survivors, the cumulative incidence of AF was more than 50%. Patients with AF had twice the chance of death [60].

In a geriatric institute, 77 geriatric patients with an average age of 80 ± 7 years, anticoagulated with warfarin and DOACs, were retrospectively enrolled after a

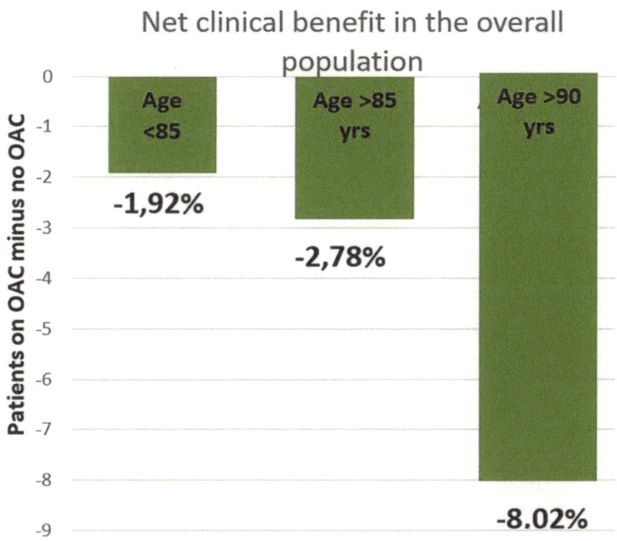

Figure 7.
Net clinical benefit adjusted for the mortality risk, of OAC vs. no OAC (adapted).

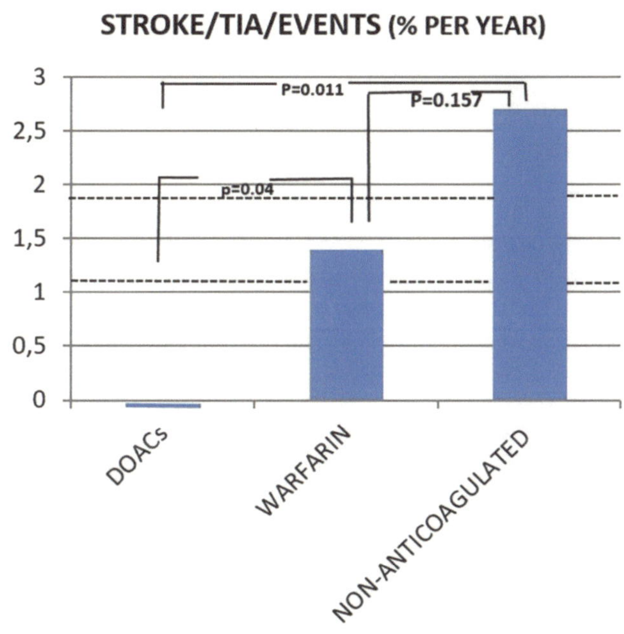

Figure 8.
Annual STROKE and TIA events.

fall from their own height or less. After admission to the hospital, he/she had a brain CT scan where the tomography image was accepted as positive if an ICH was observed.

The first brain CT had 20.8% positivity, then in an average control of 8 hours, in those patients with images that were negative, 9.8% HIC was found not detected previously.

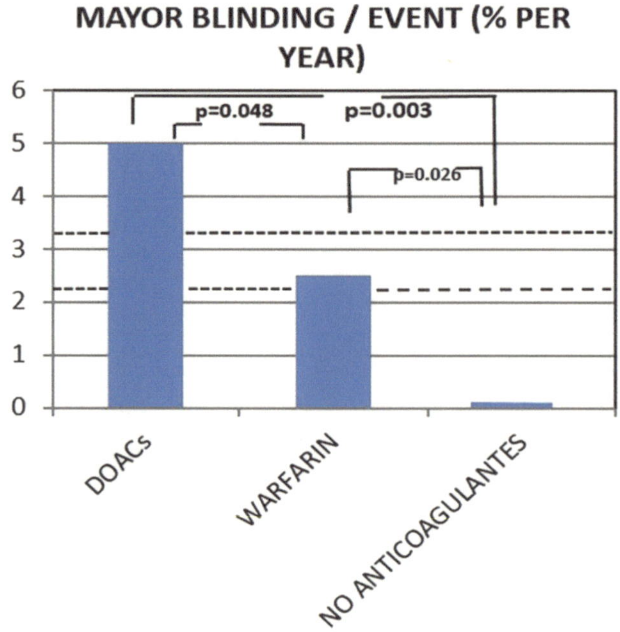

Figure 9.
Annual major bleeding events.

In the group of patients who took warfarin, there was 30% HIC vs. 14% of those who took DOACs. Patients who used DOACs had a higher rate of use of aspirin and clopidogrel [61].

In the Japanese study on anticoagulated elderly people, SAKURA-AF Registry, three groups of elderly people were enrolled, the third group, of very elderly with an average age of 87.3 years ± 2.5 (>85 years of age and under <97 years of age) where the use of DOACs and warfarin were compared.

About 45.8% DOACs were used and of these, 79% were in low doses. The study described those embolic events increase, in proportion, more than hemorrhagic events, and suggested the effective use of DOACs in very old people [62].

In a larger prevalence study of nonagenarian patients with anticoagulated AF made in the city of Madrid, published 2019, 10,077 nonagenarians (17%) had a high prevalence of comorbidities, 67.2% were anticoagulated; they used 11.6% DOACs [63].

The Berlin Registry ≥89 years studied by Wutzler et al., with an average age of 92-year-old patients who received anticoagulants by 26.5%; they used 21.1% vitamin K antagonist, and 5.4% used DOACs [64].

Regarding the falls, very frequently in nonagenarian, with the classic analysis of the Markov model, it was shown that to suffer from a dreaded subdural hematoma in anticoagulated patients with warfarin over 1 year, a hypothetical number of 295 falls is needed, to overcome the benefit of said anticoagulation [65].

When studied in patients aged 90 years old vs. <60 years old, fall mortality increases considerably (5.5% vs. 0.9%).

In a 10-year retrospective cohort study, which included 5088 traumatized patients, young and nonagenarian patients were compared.

It was observed that the <60 years had an early home discharge of 73.7% vs. 18.2% ($p < 0.001$). Patients who used aspirin had greater intracerebral bleeding ($p = 0.001$).

As for mortality caused by all injuries caused by trauma, added to death from cerebral hemorrhage, aspirin ($p = 0.046$) and warfarin ($p = <0.001$) show worse rates [66].

In the population analyzed in Spain in patients over 90 years of age in acute renal failure, the functional decline was the most frequent cause, presenting with 71% of hypertensive patients, 43% chronic kidney disease, 26% with AF among others [67].

A Korean database under review (n = 20,575) was used, where the use of DOACs and warfarin in elderly people with AF was compared.

In the total group of patients over 80 years of age, a positive benefit was observed on the outcomes of the clinical combination (ischemia, stroke and major bleeding), but there were no significant differences in people over 90 years of age; however, the largest East Asian study showed that extremely elderly patients (≥ 90 years (n=2142)), who were anticoagulated with NOACs, had benefits over the use of Warfarin.

Treatment with NOACs was preferred (83.3%), and warfarin was also used (almost 16%); of the total number of patients taking NOACs, 80% used low doses of anticoagulants [68].

GFR is extremely important in nonagenarians and we must keep in mind the Crockroft-Gaul formula for anticoagulation, it is of the simple and practical equation that contemplates a wide age range (25–100 years) [11].

Taking into account that renal function declines in elderly people, especially GFR and effective glomerular flow, with a 10% drop in the latter per milliliter/minute/body surface [69].

5. Conclusions

Over the years, patients with AF, the elderly, the very elderly, and the fragile increase the likelihood of thromboembolic diseases, as well as having bleeding with gastrointestinal predominance, after a stroke or after falls.

Since the appearance of DOACs, an optimal, versatile, and easy-to-use treatment has been found to maintain the thin balance between patients who most need to be prevented from SE and Stroke, and bleeding.

A reduction given by the drug group was obtained, an average of about 50% of HICs with a decrease in major bleeding, including GI.

The decision of the type of DOACs must be made to the measure of each patient and taking into account the precautions of a prior comprehensive assessment of the long-lived person.

Acknowledgements

To the University Professor Llopis Maria Elizabeth, Ortigoza Facundo Daniel, Ortigoza Lorenzo Tomas, and the Language Teacher E. Giaccone Diana.

Conflict of interest

The author declares no conflict of interest.

Author details

Ortigoza Daniel Víctor[1,2]

1 Committee on Arrhythmias and Electrophysiology of the Argentine Federation of Cardiology (AFC), Argentina

2 Medical Emergencies of the Lebanese Syrian Hospital, Buenos Aires, Argentina

*Address all correspondence to: dortigoza@yahoo.com.ar

References

[1] Connolly SJ, Ezekowitz MD, Yusuf F, et al. Dabigatran versus warfarin in patients with atrial fibrillation. The New England Journal of Medicine. 2009;**361**(12):1139-1151. DOI: 10.1056/NEJMoa0905561

[2] Patel M, Mahaffey K, Garg J, et al. Rivaroxaban versus warfarin in nonvalvular atrial fibrillations. The New England Journal of Medicine. 2011;**365**(10):883-889. DOI: 10.1056/NEJMoa1009638

[3] Granger C, Alexander J, McMurray J, et al. Apixaban versus warfarin in patients with atrial fibrillation. The New England Journal of Medicine. 2011;**365**:981-992. DOI: 10.1056/NEJMoa1107039

[4] Giugliano R, Ruff CT, Braunwald E, et al. Edoxaban versus warfarina in patients with atrial fibrillation. The New England Journal of Medicine. 2013;**369**(22):2093-2104. DOI: 10.1056/NEJMoa1310907

[5] Europece PMC Funders Group Author Manuscript. Frailty and the older people. Lancet. 2013;**381**(9868):752-756. DOI: 10.1016/S0140-6736(12)62167-9

[6] Hindricks G, Potpara T, Dagres N, et al. Sobre el diagnóstico y tratamiento de la fibrilación auricular, desarrollada en colaboración de la. European Association of Cardio-Thoracic Surgery (EACTS) 2021. 2020;**74**(5):378-8310. DOI: 10.1093/eurheartj/ehaa612

[7] Fauchier L, Philippart R, Clementy N, et al. How to define valvular atrial fibrillation? Archives of Cardiovascular Diseases. 2015;**108**(10):530-539. DOI: 10.1016/j.acvd.2015.06.002

[8] Deirdre A, Lip G. Use of the CHA_2DS_2-VASc and HAS-BLED scores to aid decision making for thromboprophylaxis in nonvalvular atrial fibrillation. Circulation. 2012;**126**(7):860-865. DOI: 10.1161/CIRCULACIÓN AHA.111.060061

[9] Stefell J, Collins R, Antz M, et al. European heart rhythm association practical guide on the use of non-vitamin k antagonist oral anticoagulants in patients with atrial fibrillation. EP Europace. 2021;**23**(10):1612-1676. DOI: 10.1093/europace/euab065

[10] Lip GYH, Frison L, Halperin JL, Lane CD. Comparative validation of a Novel risk score for predicting bleeding risk min anticoagulated patients with atrial fibrillation. The HAS-BLED (hypertension, abnormal renal/liver function, stroke, bleeding history or predisposition, labile INR, elderly, drugs/alcohol concomitantly) Score. Journal of the American College of Cardiology. 2011;**57**:173-180. DOI: 10.1016/j.jacc.2010.09.024

[11] Cockroft DW, Gault MH. Prediction of creatinine clearance fronserun creatinine. Nephron. 1976;**16**(1):31-41. DOI: 10.1159/000180580

[12] Fehrman-Ekholm I, Skeppholm L. Renal function in the elderly (>70 years old) measured by means of iohexol clearance, serum creatinine, serum urea and estimated clearance. Scandinavian Journal of Urology and Nephrology. 2004;**38**(1):73-77. DOI: 10.1080/00365590310015750

[13] Sukumar S, Gulilat M, Lintm B, et al. Apixabán concentrations with lower than recommended dosing in older adults with atrial fibrillation.

Journal of the American Geriatrics Society. 2019;**67**(9):1902-1906. DOI: 10.1111/jgs.15982

[14] Durand M, Schnitzer M, Pang M, et al. Effectiveness and safety among direct oral anticoagulants in nonvalvular atrial fibrillation: A multi-database cohort study with meta-analysis. British Journal of Clinical Pharmacology. 2021;**87**(6):2589-2601. DOI: 10.1111/bcp.14669

[15] Lauw MN, Eikelboom JW, Coppens M, et al. Effects of dabigatran according to age in atrial fibrillation. Heart. 2017;**103**(13):1015-1023

[16] Yavelov IS. Rivaroxaban in prevention of stroke in elderly patients with non-valvular atrial fibrillation. Kardiologiia. 2019;**59**(12S):4-11. DOI: 10.18087/cardio.n892

[17] Sadlon AH, Tsakiris DA. Direct oral anticoagulants in the elderly: Systematic review and meta-analysis of evidence, current and future directions. Swiss Medical Weekly. 2016;**146**:w14356. DOI: 10.4414/smw.2016.14356

[18] Rutherford O-CW, Jonasson C, Ghanima W, et al. Effectiveness and safety of oral anticoagulants in elderly patients with atrial fibrillation. Heart. 2021;**0**:1-8. DOI: 10.1136/heartjnl-2020-318753

[19] Kato ET, Guigliano R, Ruff C, et al. Efficacy and safety of edoxaban in elderly patients with atrial fibrillation in the ENGAGE AF–TIMI 48 trial. Journal of the American Heart Association. 2016;**5**(5):e003432. DOI: 10.1161/JAHA.116.003432

[20] Antonucci E, Poli D, Tossetto A, et al. The Italian START-register on anticoagulation with focus on atrial fibrillation. PLoS One. 2015;**10**(5):e0124719. DOI: 10.1371/journal.pone.0124719

[21] Valdiviso JM. Calcificacionvascular: Tipos y mecanismos. Nefrología (Madr.). 2011;**31**(2):1-9. Available from: http://scielo.isciii.es/scielo.php? script=sci_arttext&pid=S0211-69952011000200005

[22] Higdon J. Linus Pauling Institute. Oregon State University. Vitamin K. Available from: https://lpi.oregonstate.edu/es/mic/vitaminas/vitamina-K

[23] Huang H, Liu P, Hsu J, et al. Risk of osteoporosis in patients with atrial fibrillation using non-vitamin K antagonist oral anticoagulants or warfarin. JAHA. 2020;**9**:e013845. DOI: 10.1161/JAHA.119.013845

[24] Conen D. Epidemiology of atrial fibrillation. European Heart Journal. 2018;**39**(16):1323-1324. DOI: 10.1093/eurheartj/ehy171

[25] Figueiredo Da Mata F, Pérez Da Silva Pereira P, Cordeiro de Andrade K, et al. Prevalence of frailty in American and the Caribbean: A systematic review and meta-analysis. 2016;**11**(8):(1-8). DOI: 10.1371/journal.pone.0160019

[26] Kannel WB, Abbott RD, Savage DD, et al. Epidemiologic features of chronic atrial fibrillation: The Framingham study. The New England Journal of Medicine. 1982;**306**(17):1018-1022. DOI: 10.1056/NEJM198204293061703

[27] Carlson M, Waldo A. Fibrilación y Aleteo Auricular. In: González Zuelgaray J, editor. Arritmias Cardíacas. Buenos Aires: Inter-Médica; 1996. pp. 101-111. Chapter 6

[28] Go S, Hylek EM, Phillips KA, et al. Prevalence of diagnosed atrial fibrillation in adults: National implications for rhythm management and stroke

prevention: The anticoagulation and risk factors in atrial fibrillation (ATRIA) study. JAMA. 2001;**285**(18):2370-2375. DOI: 10.1001/jama.285.18.2370

[29] Gou Q et al. Atrial fibrillation and frailty. Journal of Geriatric Cardiology. 2020;**17**(29):105-109. DOI: 1011909/j.issn.1671-5411.202002.007

[30] Collard RM, Boter H, Scoevers R, et al. Prevalence of frailty in community-dwelling older persons: A systematic review. Journal of the American Geriatrics Society. 2012;**60**(8):1487-1492. DOI: 10.1111/j.1532-5415.2012.04054.x

[31] Staek L, Wang B, Preys S, et al. Lifetime risk of atrial fibrillation according to optimal, borderline, or elevated levels of risk factors: Cohort study based on longitudinal data from the Framingham Heart Study. BMJ Clinical Research. 2018;**361**:k1453. DOI: 10.1136/bmj.k1453

[32] Hindricks G, Potpara T, Dares N, et al. 2020 ESC Guidelines for the diagnosis and management of atrial fibrillation developed in collaboration with the European Association for Cardio-Thoracic Surgery (EACTS): The task force for the diagnosis and management of atrial fibrillation of the European Society of Cardiology (ESC) Developed with the special contribution of the European Heart Rhythm Association (EHRA) of the ESC. European Heart Journal. 2021;**42**(5):373-498. DOI: 10.1093/eurheartj/ehaa612

[33] Fried L, Ferrucci L, Derer J, et al. Untangling the concepts of disability, frailty and comorbidity: Implications for improved targeting and care. The Journals of Gerontology. Series A, Biological Sciences and Medical Sciences. 2004;**59**(3):255-263. DOI: 10.1093/gerona/59.3.m255

[34] Ortigoza D, Valentino M. Uso non-vitamin K Antagonists in frail patients with atrial fibrillation. Revista de la Federacion Argentina de Cardiologia. 2021;**50**(2):43-48. Available from: https://revistafac.org.ar/ojs/index.php/revistafac/issue/view/11

[35] Tiedemann A, Lord S, Sherrington C. The development and validation of a brief performance-based fall risk assessment tool for use in primary care. The Journals of Gerontology. Series A, Biological Sciences and Medical Sciences. 2010;**65**(8):896-903. DOI: 10.1093/gerona/glq067

[36] El Anciano frágil y riesgo nutricional. Available from: https://www.nutricionemocional.es/sites/default/files/infogeriatria_n16_final_1.pdf

[37] Oliveras Santos P, Soares da Siva I, Araújo S. Functional capacity of elderly people attending the family health program at Viveiros, Feira de Santana, Bahia, Brazil. Acta Fisiatrica. 2012;**19**(4):233-236. DOI: 10.5935/0104-7795.20120037D

[38] Chalson M, Pompei P, Ales K, et al. A new method of classifying prognostic comorbidity in longitudinal studies: Development and validation. Journal of Chronic Diseases. 1987;**40**(5):373-383. DOI: 10.1016/0021-9681(87)90171-8

[39] Peterson JC, Paget SA, Lachs MS, et al. The risk of comorbility. Annals of the Rheumatic Diseases. 2012;**71**:635-637. DOI: 10.1136/annrheumdis-2011-200473

[40] Fried LP, Tangen CM, Walston J, et al. Frailty in older adults: Evidence for a phenotype. The Journals of Gerontology, Series A: Biological Sciences. 2001;**56**(3):M146-M156. DOI: 10.1093/gerona/56.3.m146

[41] Rockwood K, Song X, MacKnight C, et al. A global clinical measure of fitness and 40-frailty in elderly people. CMAJ.

2005;**173**(5):489-495. DOI: 10.1503/cmaj.050051

[42] Ortigoza D, Taranto L. The attention system in a hospital's emergency medical service. Salud(i)Ciencia. 2019;**23**(6):519-523. DOI: 10.21840/siic/160015. Available from: https://www.siicsalud.com/dato/sic/236/160015.pdf

[43] Fumagalli S, Potpara TS, Bjerregaard Larsen T, et al. Frailty syndrome: An emerging clinical problem in the everyday management of clinical arrhythmias. The results of the European Heart Rhythm Association survey. EP Europace. 2017;**19**(11):1896-1902. DOI: 10.1093/europace/eux288

[44] Patti G, Mantione L, Bressi E, et al. Efficacy and safety of oral anticoagulant therapy in frail patients with atrial fibrillation. Monaldi Archives for Chest Disease. 2018;**88**(2):10-12. DOI: 10.4081/monaldi.2018.958

[45] Rao M, Vinereanu D, Wojdyla D, et al. Clinical outcomes and history of fall in patients with atrial fibrillations treated with oral anticoagulation: Insights from the ARISTOTLE trial. The American Journal of Medicine. 2018;**131**(3):269-275. DOI: 10.1016/j.amjmed.2017.10.036

[46] Steffel J, Gugliano RP, Braunwald E, Murphy S, et al. Edoxaban versus warfarina; in atrial fibrillation patients at risk of falling. ENANGE AF-TIM 48 analysis. Journal of the American College of Cardiology. 2016;**68**:1169-1178. DOI: 10.1016/j.jacc.2016.06.034

[47] Lip G, Keshishian A, Kang A, Damane A, et al. Oral anticoagulants for nonvalvular atrial fibrillation in frail elderly patients: Insights from the ARISTOPHANES study. Journal of Internal Medicine. 2021;**289**(1):42-52. DOI: 10.1111/joim.13140

[48] Hanon O, Chaussade E, David JP, et al. SAFIR cohort: One-year prospective follow-up of very old and frail patients treated with direct oral anticoagulant, rivaroxaban. Archives of Cardiovascular Diseases Supplements. 2020;**12**(1):115. DOI: 10.1016/j.acvdsp.2019.09.250

[49] Bauersachs RM, Herold J. Oral anticoagulation in the elderly and frail. Hämostaseologie. 2020;**40**:74-83. DOI: 10.1055/s-0040-1701476

[50] Población residente por fecha, sexo y edad. Total Nacional (90 años y más). Instituto nacional de estadística INE; 2021. Available from: https://www.ine.es/jaxiT3/Tabla.htm?t=31304

[51] Instituto Nacional de Estadística y Censos de la República Argentina. Población y estimaciones (90 años y más). Available from: https://www.indec.gob.ar/indec/web/Nivel4-Tema-2-24-84

[52] Bevölkerung in absolutenZahlen, Anteile der Altersgruppen in Prozent, 1960 bis 2050 StatistischesBundesamt: Lange Reihen: Bevölkerungnach Altersgruppen, 13. koordinierte Bevölkerungsvorausberechnung: BevölkerungDeutschlandsbis 2060: BundeszentralefürPolitischeBildung. Available from: https://www.bpb.de/nachschlagen/zahlen-und-fakten/soziale-situation-in-deutschland/61541/altersstruktur

[53] Lernfelt G, Mandalenakis Z, Hornestam B, et al. Atrial fibrillation in the ederly general population: A 30-years follow-up from 70 to 100 years of age. Scandinavian Cardiovascular Journal. 2020;**54**(4):232-238. DOI: 10.1080/14017431.2020.1729399

[54] Kodani E, Atarashi H, Inoue H, Okumura K, Yamashita T, Origasa H. Use of warfarin in elderly patients

with non-valvular atrial fibrillation—subanalysis of the J-RHYTHM registry. Circulation Journal. 2015;**79**(11):2345-2352. DOI: 10.1253/circj.cj-15-0621

[55] Chao T-F, Chiang C-E, Chan Y-H, et al. Oral anticoagulants in extremely-high-risk, very elderly (>90 years) patients with atrial fibrillation. Heart Rhythm. 2021;**18**(6):871-877. DOI: 10.1016/j.hrthm.2021.02.018

[56] Raposeiras-Roubín S, Rodríguez DA, Freire SJC. Vitamin K antagonists and direct oral anticoagulants in nonagenarian patients with atrial fibrillation. DOI: 10.1016/j.jamda.2019.08.033. Epub 2019 Nov 19, 1-7

[57] Patti G, Lucerna M, Pecen L, Siller-Matula JM, Cavallari I, Kirchhof P, et al. Thromboembolic risk, bleeding outcomes and efect of diferent antithrombotic strategies in very elderly patients with atrial fibrillation: A sub-analysis from the PREFER in AF (PREvention oF thromboembolic events-european registry in atrial fbrillation). Journal of the American Heart Association. 2017;**6**:e005657. DOI: 10.1161/JAHA.117.005657

[58] Yamaji H, Higashiya S, Murakami T. Effects of oral anticoagulants on patients with atrial fibrillation aged 90 years and older: Comparison among direct oral anticoagulant, warfarin anticoagulant, and nonanticoagulation. Journal of Cardiovascular Pharmacology. 2019;**74**:246-245. DOI: 10.1097/FJC.0000000000000703

[59] Poli D, Antonucci E, Ageno W, Bertù L, Migliaccio L, Martinese L, et al. Oral anticoagulation in very elderly patients with atrial fibrillation: Results from the prospective multicenter START2-REGISTER study. PLoS One. 2019;**14**(5):e0216831. DOI: 10.1371/journal.pone.0216831

[60] Lernfelt G, Mandalenakis Z, Hornestam B, et al. Atrial fibrillation in the elderly general population: A 30-year follow-up from 70 to 100 years of age. Scandinavian Cardiovascular Journal. 2020;**54**(4):232-238. DOI: 10.1080/14017431.2020.1729399

[61] Cocca A, Privette A, Leon S, et al. Delayed intracranial hemorrhage in anticoagulated geriatric patients after ground level falls. The Journal of Emergency Medicine. 2019;**57**(6):812-816. DOI: 10.1016/j.jemermed.2019.09.011

[62] Nishida T, Okumura Y, Yokoyama K, et al. Oral anticoagulant use and clinical outcomes in elderly Japanese patients: Findings from the SAKURA AF registry. Heart and Vessels. 2019;**34**(12):2021-2030. DOI: 10.1007/s00380-019-01446-6

[63] Lahoz C, Cárdenas J, Salinero-Ford M, et al. Prevalence of atrial fibrillation and associated anticoagulant therapy in the nonagenarian population of the Community of Madrid, Spain. Geriatrics & Gerontology International. 2019;**19**(3):203-207. DOI: 10.1111/ggi.13587

[64] Wutzler A, von Ulmenstein S, Attanasio P, et al. Treatment of nonagenarians with atrial fibrillation: Insights from the Berlin atrial fibrillation (BAF) registry. Journal of the American Medical Directors Association;**16**(11):969-972. DOI: 10.1016/j.jamda.2015.05.012

[65] Man-Son-Hing M, Nichol G, Lau A, Laupacis A. Choosing antithrombotic therapy for elderly patients with atrial fibrillation who are at risk for falls. 1999;**159**(7):677-685. DOI: 10.1001/archinte.159.7.677

[66] Bhattacharya B, Maung A, Schuster K, Kimberly A, et al. The

older they are the harder they fall: Injury patterns and outcomes by age after ground level falls. Injury. 2016;**47**(9):1955-1959. DOI: 10.1016/j.injury.2016.06.019

[67] Begoña S, Sanz M, Muños Ramos P, et al. Baseline characteristics of nonagenarians hospitalised due to acute kidney injury compared to other age groups. Revista Española de Geriatría y Gerontología. 2020;**55**(6):326-331. DOI: 10.1016/j.regg.2020.06.004

[68] Kwon S, So-R L, Choi EK, et al. Non-vitamin K antagonist oral anticoaulantsinveryederly east Asians with atrial fibrillation: A nationwide population-based Study. American Heart Journal. 2020;**229**:81-91. DOI: 10.1016/j.ahj.2020.08.006

[69] Musso C, Oreopoulos D. Aging and physiological changes of the kidneys including changes in glomerular filtration rate. Nephron. Physiology. 2011;**119**(Suppl. 1):1-p5. DOI: 10.1159/000328010

Chapter 4

Danaparoid Sodium: A Review of Its Use in Hepatic Thrombotic Disorders

Harry N. Magnani

Abstract

Danaparoid sodium is an antithrombotic isolated from porcine mucosa. Its main constituent is a mixture of heparan sulphates that inhibits thrombin generation and also possesses anti-inflammatory and immune-modulatory activity. It has shown safety and efficacy in its main indications of deep venous thrombosis prophylaxis, heparin-induced thrombocytopenia treatment and disseminated intravascular thrombosis treatment. In addition, there are reports of its off-label use for the treatment of portal vein thrombosis in adults and for prevention of the hepatic thrombotic microangiopathies haematogenous that complicate recovery after stem cell transplantation in adults and children. The results of these studies provide further support for its safety and efficacy even in subjects with cirrhosis and/or severe hepatic dysfunction. In this chapter the rationale for danaparoid use is presented and the collated results of comparative studies and case reports are compared with those of other pharmaceutical options for managing these hepatic thrombotic disorders.

Keywords: danaparoid, PVT, SOS, TA-TMA, HSCT, hepatic thromboses

1. Introduction

The liver is the largest organ in the body, and while it only accounts for about 3% of the total body weight it receives 25% [1, 2] of the cardiac output via the hepatic artery and portal vein. This is due to its multifunctionality in regulating glucose and amino acid homeostasis, detoxifying the blood, processing of lipoproteins and their fats, synthesis of bile and proteins, storage of glycogen and vitamins and filtering of bacteria, etc.

Hepatocytes produce many of the proteins involved in normal regulation of the clotting cascade and fibrinolytic system. These, with platelets, achieve a balanced haemostasis system with fine controls and checks at many levels to maintain free flow of blood within the circulation, prevent uncontrolled clotting of the blood and quickly plug blood vessel wall breaches to limit blood loss. Toxins and pathogens can not only cause hepatocyte injury but also damage hepatic sinusoidal cells and endothelial cells (ECs) throughout the circulation. The injury results in reduced synthesis of clotting factors but due to compensating changes in additional factors that regulate the clotting and fibrinolytic cascades, haemostasis and thrombin generation remain in balance [3] and any bleeding is usually due to the presence of varices. This new haemostasis balance is more sensitive to perturbation because synthesis and release of proteins and proteases responsible for its fine tuning, that come not only from hepatocytes but also sinusoidal cells and ECs, are also disrupted. The initial result is more likely to be a procoagulant state, but if hepatic dysfunction worsens the balance may tip the other way with predomination of fibrinolysis, thrombocytopenia and worsening platelet dysfunction causing bleeding.

2. Portal vein thrombosis

The haemostasis disruption may lead to macro-vascular thromboses involving the complex circulation around the liver, i.e. the portal venous system (PVS) that includes the intra-hepatic portal vein branches, the splenic and superior mesenteric veins. Portal vein thrombosis (PVT) commonly occurs in patients with hepatic cirrhosis and/or carcinoma, while splenic vein thrombosis may also be found as an extension of a PVT or develop as a complication of splenectomy [4, 5]. PVT may also develop in the absence of primary liver disease [6] and has recently been described in patients with COVID-19 [7, 8] and in patients suffering vaccine-induced immune thrombocytopenic thrombosis (VITT) following COVID-19 vaccination [9].

In patients with cirrhosis the frequency of PVT increases with disease severity [10] from about 3%–25% [11]. In post-splenectomy patients with cirrhosis the frequency may reach 36% in the absence of anticoagulation and rates as high as 70%–5% have been found in the presence of malignancy (hepatoma, lymphomas, solid tumours, myeloproliferative neoplasms). Although at first PVT may be almost symptomless and many spontaneously disappear, persistence and recurrence result in significant or complete obstruction of one or more vessels of the PVS and portal hypertension with increasing morbidity. Formation of collateral circulations and varices are prone to rupture with often major blood loss. PVT can present either acutely with abdominal pain, diarrhoea and ileus—occasionally as an acute abdomen or chronically often with signs of portal hypertension.

Persistent/recurrent PVS thrombosis (PVST) may eventually be fatal, hence there is frequently a need for effective antithrombotic management. Especially if acute non-occlusive PVST or a thrombotic risk factor is present, e.g. sepsis, cancer, antiphospholipid antibody or an acquired or hereditary thrombotic risk (factor V Leiden, prothrombin mutation G20210A, protein C and/or S deficiency, etc.) then anticoagulation should be considered [12, 13]. The aims of anticoagulation are thrombus recanalisation, reduction of portal hypertension to lower the bleeding risk and prevention of PVST recurrence. The use of anticoagulants has been reviewed and several meta-analyses of the results are available [5, 14]. Despite the heterogeneity of the included studies, there appears to be a growing consensus that use of anticoagulants for the treatment of PVT increases the rate of recanalisation compared with non-anticoagulated patients, but there is too little evidence concerning their benefit to risk balance with emphasis on bleeding complications.

3. Sinusoidal obstruction syndrome and transplant associated thrombotic microangiopathy

The sinusoidal cells, which share many features of ECs, are particularly at risk of toxic injury. Both hepatic sinusoidal obstruction syndrome (SOS) and transplant associated thrombotic microangiopathy (TA-TMA) are examples of sinusoidal cell and EC injury. Detoxification of chemotherapeutic drugs and other toxins, including pathogen induced endotoxins, is mediated by the hepatic cytochrome P450 complex and any toxic side-products produced are neutralised by the glutathione enzymatic system (GSH). The centrilobular cells of the sinusoids have the least GSH and the lowest oxygen supply thus they are at most risk of toxic injury. If the activity of the P450 and/or GSH is impaired or overwhelmed, e.g. in hepatic disorders and/or the presence of high intensity chemotherapy, then toxic side-products accumulate leading to sinusoidal and EC injury. The resultant disruption of local haemostasis and immune system control result in microvascular thromboses the development of SOS [15] (formerly known as veno occlusive disease or VOD). The injury may extend beyond the sinusoids allowing toxic chemotherapeutic drugs and their side products to access ECs in the general circulation and other organs. If these are already injured by prior total body radiation and/or infections or by graft v host disease (GvHD) following haematogenous stem cell transplantation (HSCT), then further endothelial damage will develop with gradual or sudden emergence of the clinical and pathological picture of TA-TMA. Both SOS and TA-TMA occur most frequently as complications of HSCT as a result of the chemotherapy used to prepare for the transplant, the use of allogeneic in place of autologous transplants and post-transplant use of further chemotherapy and a cocktail of drugs to prevent or control infection, transplant rejection and GvHD. Both SOS and TA-TMA are associated with a high mortality. **Table 1** shows risk factor associated with one or both complications.

Complement cascade proteins also originate in the liver. In health the immunological/anti-inflammatory and haemostatic systems are finely tuned and, because of their cross-talk via various interacting pathways, maintain a finely balanced vascular homeostasis ready to repel 'foreign' invasion and seal damaged vessels to limit blood loss and procoagulant products (including PAI-1, thrombomodulin, vWF and microparticles). However, sinusoidal cell and EC injury related to HSCT injury leads to release of a cocktail of cytokines and mitogens, the so-called 'cytokine storm'. Unregulated complement activation [16–20] ensues and the balance and cross-talk between haemostasis and the immune systems is disturbed. The result is further EC damage with fibrin deposition and thrombi feeding into the pathogenesis of both SOS and TA-TMA.

SOS usually manifests within 21 days but may present late, with thrombocytopenia and signs of portal hypertension due to fibrous obliteration of the sinusoids and central venules. Endothelial injury underlies both disorders but for some [21] this is insufficient to consider SOS as a vascular endothelial syndrome. However, others [22] disagree since TA-TMA, with its mixed endothelial/immune origin is included [21]. Furthermore, immunological involvement in the pathogenesis of SOS is also very likely since injured ECs release cytokines and mitogens and these are capable of complement cascade activation and disruption [23]. These can also activate the coagulation cascade via the intrinsic pathway further increasing thrombin production. Observations that the frequency of SOS increases with the use of mis-matched and unrelated donor cells and is redusced in T-cell depleted HSCT also point to an immunological connection. The overall frequency of SOS development after bone-marrow transplantation (BMT) is about 14% (range 5%–50%), depending upon the chemotherapeutic drug and/or conditioning regimen used for cancer treatment and transplantation, and the clinical diagnostic criteria used [24, 25]. Children appear to be more prone to SOS but the wide range is greatly influenced by diagnostic imprecision, clinical status of the patient at BMT, and the conditions of the transplant, particularly the type of conditioning used. SOS is associated with a 40% mortality but in the presence of organ disfunction this may rise to 80%.

Risk factor cited for occurrence and severity	SOS	TA-TMA
Gender (F > M)		(+)
Age at HSCT <10 years	+	
Use of: alkylating cytostatic agents, platinum complexed agents, pyrrolizidine plant alkaloids	+	+
Immunotherapies for acute leukaemias: gemtuzumab, inotuzumab, ozogamicin,	+	+
Donor mismatch		+
Platelet transfusion mismatch	+	
Number of prior stem-cell transplants		+
Fungal or viral infections/sepsis		+
Pre-existing hepatic injury (viral, cancer)	+	
Active co-morbidity		+
Prior abdominal radiotherapy	+	+
Immunodeficiency syndrome		+
Presence of an autoimmune disorder		+
The interval between malignancy diagnosis and the HSCT	+	
Presence of acute GvHD		+
Inherited thrombophilia (FVL, G20210A)		+
Post HSCT cyclosporine, tacrolimus, serolimus		+
After autologous as well as allogeneic BMT	(+)	(+)
Liver transplantation	+	

Table 1.
Risk factors for SOS and TA-TMA.

TA-TMA usually presents at any time within the first 3 months of transplantation but may appear up to several years after the HSCT. The overall frequency of TA-TMA is about 5% but up to 76% [26] has been reported (see **Table 1**). Mortality may reach 80% and is related to the number of risk factors present, e.g. the type of cytotoxic agent, particularly methotrexate, cyclophosphamide, etc., used in the conditioning regimens for transplantation, presence of active infection, use of matched unrelated donors, transplant mismatches, presence of GvHD and previous BMT. Survivors may suffer long term morbidity due to chronic organ damage.

Perhaps TA-TMA represents a vascular form of GvHD since it may precede the appearance of GvHD and its frequency increases with the severity of GvHD [21] and they share similarities in pathophysiology [27–29]. These considerations may explain the overlaps and differences between SOS and TA-TMA in their risk factors (see **Table 1**) and their distribution, clinical presentation and sequelae (see **Table 2**). In addition, it may account for their presence together in some patients and the continuing controversy over their diagnostic criteria that confounds early recognition and treatment of both disorders.

It is possible that SOS and TA-TMA are different clinical presentations of the same problem. Their pathogenesis is similar and the resulting sinusoidal and EC injury triggers release of many factors resulting in disruption of both haemostasis and immune systems. In this respect both SOS and TA-TMA are similar to the general group of microangiopathies [22, 30].

Reported disease characteristics[1]	**SOS**	**TA-TMA**
Frequency	2%–60%	5%–20%
Post HSCT onset:		
Adults acute	<21 days	No limit (1–3 months)
Adults chronic	≥21 days	
Paediatric	No limit	
Frequency:		
Adults	≥40%	About 8%
Paediatrics	≥17%	
Organ dysfunction:		
Liver	+	+
Kidney	+	+
Lung	+	+
GI tract	–	+
CNS problems	+	Late
Cardiac	–	+
Polyserositis	–	+
MOD	early	+
Fluid retention	+	+
Hypertension	—	+
Laboratory:		
Thrombocytopenia	+	+
Haemolytic anaemia	–	+
Schistocytes	–	+
Lactate dehydrogenase	–	+
Indirect and direct Coomb's tests	—	+
Complement activation	(+)	+
Pro-inflammatory markers	TNFα, ICAM-1	TNFα, VCAM-1
Haemostasis impairment	vWF, TM, PAI-1	vWF, TM
Mortality	5% (1–>60%)[1]	40–>80%

[1]*Depending upon the rapidity with which the clinical status worsens and time of assessment.*

Table 2.
Some characteristics of SOS and TA-TMA after HSCT compared.

It is clear that both antithrombotic and immune modulating drugs are indicated to prevent or treat both conditions. However, prevention is always better than cure if the right product is available. The ability of a single product to attenuate the effects of both systems without causing further damage would be a desirable bonus especially if this can be done safely and relatively cheaply.

4. Danaparoid

Danaparoid sodium is a mixture of linear glycosaminoglycuronans (GAGs) with a MW_{ave} of 4500 Da (range 2500–10,000 Da). It is extracted from porcine mucosa after heparin removal and ultrafiltration. The final product consists of heparan sulphate (HS) 85% with about 12% dermatan sulphate (DS) and traces of chondroitin sulphates 4 and 6 (CS). The HS appears to be more concentrated in the lower MW_{ave} chains and the DS and CS in the longer chains. The main structural difference between danaparoid and the heparins is the presence of glucuronic acid in place of iduronic acid. Enzyme degradation of danaparoid GAG chains produces disaccharides (see **Figure 1**) with a low degree of sulphation and acidification. Hence the GAG chains in danaparoid a low overall negative charge density compared with the heparins [unfractionated (UFH) and the fractionated low molecular weight heparins (LMWHs)]. However, about 5% by weight of the HS fraction of danaparoid [the so-called high affinity HS (HA-HS)] consists of more highly sulphated chains because like those of UFH they contain an antithrombin (AT) binding pentasaccharide sequence that includes a triple sulphated glucosamine residue. Only this specific AT binding site possesses a higher overall negative surface charge density than the rest of danaparoid chains that do not bind AT.

Danaparoid is an antithrombotic that inhibits thrombin generation by both AT mediated inhibition of factor Xa by the HA-HS subfraction and direct inhibition of thrombin activation of factor IX by the major non AT binding HS. In addition, a minor inhibition of thrombin activity is produced by the HA-HS, mediated via AT, and by the DS fraction mediated via heparin-cofactor II.

Danaparoid is not a heparin but a heparinoid and further, unlike the heparins, it is not an anticoagulant because the recommended therapeutic dose regimen hardly affects the routine clotting tests (aPTT, PT, ACT and TT). A lack of spontaneous platelet activation and the weak inhibition of thrombin-induced platelet activation is associated with virtually normal primary haemostasis and hence low bleeding risk.

Three biological effects of danaparoid can be assayed—its anti-Xa activity, anti-thrombin activity and TGI. These have plasma half-lives of 24.7, 2.0 and 6.7 h respectively. However, the anti-thrombin activity is too weak for monitoring and at the time of its clinical development (1980s) there was no simple TGI assay. Hence the pharmacokinetics of danaparoid was based on the effect of the smallest subfraction

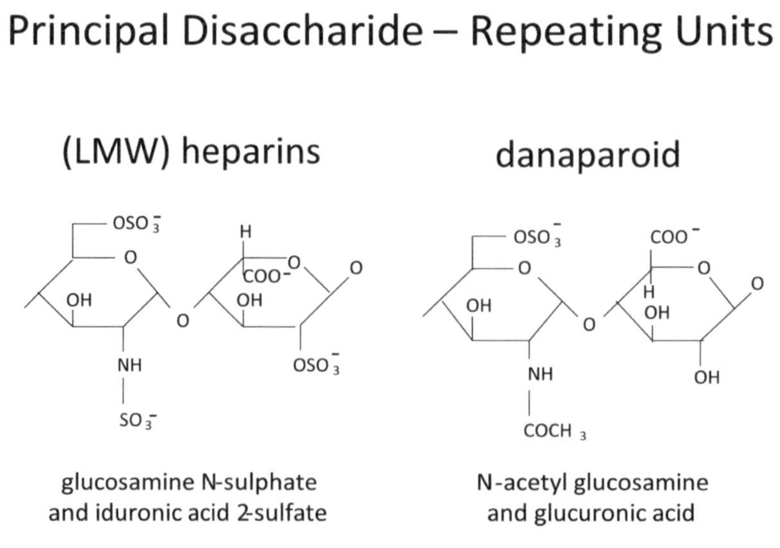

Figure 1.
Comparison of heparin and danaparoid disaccharide structures.

of danaparoid (HA-HS) that represents only 5% by weight of the total product and is responsible for only half of its anti-thrombotic activity.

Plasma anti-Xa activity measurements have shown that at least the HA-HS subfraction is cleared via the kidneys and that the liver plays no role in its elimination from the blood. In the absence of overall labelling studies it is assumed that the remaining fractions of danaparoid undergo a similar fate. Although useful for estimating plasma levels of danaparoid the anti-Xa activity shows poor correlation with bleeding or thrombotic events reflecting the fact that this assay, unlike thrombin generation inhibition (TGI), does not measure all actions contributing to danaparoid's effect on haemostasis.

Only 5% of the HS chains in danaparoid contain the trisulphated disaccharide required for AT binding. The remaining chains are low in both sulphate and acidic groups hence the overall negative charge density of danaparoid is low compared with the heparins (see **Figure 1**). Thus danaparoid is unable to bind to the many positively charged 'heparin-binding' proteins in the circulation and without this 'neutralising effect' danaparoid is 100% bioavailable for antithrombotic activity compared with 30% for UFH and about 80% for the LMWHs. This is also the reason why the anti-Xa activity units (U) of danaparoid are not equivalent to the IU of the heparins.

Clinical development of danaparoid led to widespread approval for deep venous thrombosis (DVT) prophylaxis hip following hip orthopaedic and general cancer surgery and in Japan for the treatment of disseminated intravascular thrombosis (DIC). The absence of heparin making it unlikely to cross-react with the specific antiplatelet antibody led to its approval for the treatment of heparin-induced thrombocytopenia (HIT), including the prevention or treatment of thrombosis in patients with renal failure requiring use of an extracorporeal circuits, in children and in pregnancy, if these patients also have HIT or other forms of heparin intolerance. **Table 3** compares some PK and PD aspects of danaparoid with those of the heparins.

Apart from its antithrombotic activity, animal and isolated tissue experiments revealed that like heparin danaparoid has both immune-modulatory and anti-inflammatory activities [32], with both similarities and differences from the heparins (see **Table 4**).

The first indication of this came when danaparoid prevented heparin from activating platelets in the presence of plasma from patients with HIT [33]. In addition, it was found that while the isolated HA-HS subfraction (4% by weight of danaparoid) showed 100% cross reactivity with the specific HIT antibody this was totally prevented by addition of the remaining 96% of danaparoid with no affinity for AT [34]. Finally it was shown that danaparoid is unique among currently available antithrombotics in interfering with the interactions of the specific HIT antibody with heparin and its platelet and monocyte targets [35]. In addition, it was shown that danaparoid is unable complex with platelet factor 4 (PF4, a platelet derived cytokine to which heparin binds to induce HIT) to form the ultra-high molecular weight complexes with neo-antigenic sites [36] required to induce the specific antiplatelet antibody underlying the pathogenesis of HIT. Other experiments [37–49] (summarised in **Table 4**, where it is compared with the effects of the heparins) have shown that danaparoid inhibits or attenuates anti-inflammatory effects induced by various triggers, including endotoxin, ischaemia, reduction of ischaemia/reperfusion-induced hepatic injury in animals and a pilot endotoxin study in volunteers. Many of these actions occurred at the equivalent of its usual therapeutic dosing intensities. They appear to be independent of danaparoid's antithrombotic activity, since they occur in the absence of AT or other clotting cascade constituents. From independent studies of synthetic GAGs or chemically modified heparin the resultant chemical structure of its oligosaccharide chains is of great importance. The low degree of sulphation with fewer acid groups and

	UFH	LMWH	Danaparoid
Coagulation cascade inhibition[1]:			
Co-factor dependent	IXa, Xa, XIa, IIa	Xa, IIa	Xa, [IIa]
Co-factor independent	IXa	IXa	IXa
Potency in buffer:			
Anti-Xa	193 IU/mg	80–120 IU/mg	18 U/mg
Anti-IIa	193 IU/mg	35–45 IU/mg	<1.0 U/mg
Bioavailability (IV)	20%–30%	85%–95%	~100%
Elimination half-life IV (hours)	1.5 (a-Xa)	4.0 (a-Xa)	6.7 (TGI)
Elimination route	RE system	Renal 10%–40%	Renal >50%
Administration route	IV, SC	IV, SC	IV, SC
Clotting test prolongation[2]	aPTT,PT,TT,HepT	aPTT,PT,TT,HepT	HepT only
Thrombin inhibition	Yes	Yes	Very weak
TGI	Yes	Yes	Yes
Platelet activation	Yes	Yes	No
Increase fibrinolysis	Yes	Yes	No
Increases clot permeability[3]	Yes	No	Yes
Plasma protein binding	Very high	Moderately high	[no][4]
Bleeding inducing capacity	At high doses	Low	Low
AT concentration sensitive	Yes	Yes	[no][5]
Effect on APC production	Reduces	[reduces]	Maintains
Inhibition of clot bound IIa	At very high doses	No	No

[ ] square brackets indicates action greatly reduced or virtually absent, APC = activated protein C.
[1]Roman numerals refer to clotting factors.
[2]aPTT, PT and TT measure residual thrombin activity, the HepT (Heptest) measures anti-Xa and anti-IIa activities.
[3]Increases plasmin access.
[4]Only to its specific targets: AT and HCoII.
[5]One study of PVT treatment [31] found less efficacy of dan if AT <50%.

Table 3.
The heparins and danaparoid, modes of action, pharmacokinetics and pharmacodynamics compared.

the absence of the 2-O sulphate group on the glucosamine (see **Figure 1**) appear to be responsible for many of the immune-modulatory/anti-inflammatory activities summarised in **Table 4** [31, 32, 50–53].

Thus fine structural differences between the many HSs within the body are responsible for myriad interactions that are site-specific with roles in haemostasis, inflammation, leukocyte transmigration, immune homeostasis, lipid metabolism, cell attachment, angiogenesis, migration, invasion and cell differentiation.

Based on the combination of antithrombotic activity and immune/modulatory actions danaparoid has been successfully used to treat patients with sepsis, DIC and HIT. In addition its low bleeding inducing capacity has led to off label use to prevent post-HSCT SOS and TA-TMA and to treat patients with PVT.

Inhibition or reduces:	Heparin	LMWHs	Danaparoid
Endotoxin lung injury[1]:			
Local	Yes	Yes	Yes
Coagulopathy Inflammation	No	nd	No
Fibrinolysis systemic	No	nd	No
Coagulopathy	Yes	Yes	Yes
Reperfusion injury	Yes	Yes	Yes
Anti-inflammatory	Yes	Yes	Yes
Endothelial glycocalyx damage	(yes)	(yes)	Yes
Growth factor production	Yes	Yes	Yes
Interferon	Yes	Yes	Yes
Burn/smoke inhalation injury	Yes	Yes	Yes
Endothelial injury	Yes	Yes	Yes
Intimal hyperplasia	Yes	(yes)	(yes)
Cell proliferation	Yes	Yes	Yes
Angiogenesis	Yes	Yes	Yes
Annexin binding[2]	Yes	Yes	Yes
Tissue and/or organ damage	Yes	(yes)	nd
Leucocyte activation and adhesion	Yes	Yes	Yes
NET formation	Yes	Yes	nd
Effects of HMGB-1	Yes	Yes	Yes
Immunogenic binding with PF4	Yes	Yes	No
Virus transduction	Yes	(yes)	weak[4]
Spontaneous 'HIT' induction	No	No	Yes
HIT antibody interactions	No	No	Yes

HIT = heparin-induced thrombocytopenia, HMGB-1 is a chromatin protein and cytokine mediator of inflammation, NET = neutrophil extracellular trap, PF4 = platelet factor 4.
[1]However highly dependent on the specific annexin and degree of sulphation of the GAG involved.
[2]Single report using recombinant adeno-associated virus- type 2[4].
nd—no data, brackets indicate action is weaker or only occurs under certain circumstances.

Table 4.
GAG immune-modulatory effects at therapeutic dose levels.

4.1 Danaparoid treatment of portal vein thrombosis

4.1.1 Population exposure

Danaparoid exposure in relation to PVT is available for 559 patients. Five retrospective comparative studies treated 177 patients with danaparoid only v UFH [54], v danaparoid + AT [55, 56] or v danaparoid + AT and AT only [57] and danaparoid + AT v AT only [58]. In addition, 383 patients received danaparoid in reports of retrospective case series and single case reports [57, 59–91] in which danaparoid was used alone or combined with AT and finally 2 single case reports of danaparoid administered with UFH [92] or urokinase [93]. Danaparoid was given to treat the PVT in 41 of the 43 reports. In the remaining 2 it

Parameter[1]	Danaparoid use in comparative studies			Danaparoid use in case reports[2]	
	Alone	With AT	Controls	Alone	With AT
N2	75	64	118	390	
Age (range in years)			23–85		
M/F distribution (%)	35.1/64.9				
Cirrhosis	67/67		7/7	329/355	
Varices	105/107			197/283	
Hepatocellular cancer	65/107			113/274	

AT = Antithrombin.
[1]*Not all studies had complete information hence the different denominator.*
[2]*Danaparoid was compared in most studies with danaparoid + AT. In Ref. [31] the number receiving dan alone or + AT is only specified in an interim analysis for 28 of the final 55 patients. Three additional case reports of dan + UK, dan + UFH and dan + warfarin are not included in table but are discussed in text.*

Table 5.
General characteristics of PVT of danaparoid treated patients and non-danaparoid controls.

was given for PVT prophylaxis. **Table 5** shows some patient characteristics that could be identified with the treatment given.

Hepatic PVT was present in 524 of the 558 patients exposed to danaparoid (including those receiving AT and the 3 receiving concomitant antithrombotics—UFH, warfarin or a thrombolytic). In 33 patients thrombus was also present in the splenic vein and in 33 in the superior mesenteric vein, but only 11 single case reports stated the exact distributions when 2 or more sites were implicated, i.e. PV + SMV 6 cases, PV + SV 1 case, PV + SV and SMV 3 cases and PV + B-Ch 1 case and one publication mentioned that in 16 of 41 patients the PVT was present in more than 1 site.

The frequencies of some relevant presenting parameters were inconsistently provided in the study reports, e.g. hepatic failure was hardly mentioned but one study [60] reported a mean MELD score of 8.6, encephalopathy was only mentioned in four reports, the Child-Pugh status was provided for 10 comparative studies and 6 case reports as either scores (range 5–12) or classes A, B and C—118, 166 and 49 respectively, bleeding (in all cases gastrointestinal, 3 due to varices) was only mentioned in 6 single case reports and severe infection in only 3 reports, mean plasma AT levels available in only 8 publications were low normal or <60% of normal levels in 7 and platelet counts provided in only 5 single case reports and 4 comparative studies or case series were a median 80 G/L (range 17–655). It is not known if these parameters were therefore normal, absent or not considered, hence their absence from the pooled overview shown in **Table 5**.

Patients were followed-up after danaparoid discontinuation for at least 3 months and in some studies events up to 2 or 3 years were recorded. During this follow-up period at least 210 patients had been transitioned to a warfarin to continue anticoagulation. One study [66] found that long-term edoxaban succeeded but warfarin failed to sustain successful initial danaparoid treatment of PVT.

4.1.2 Danaparoid dosing for PVT

All studies, apart from three single cases [72, 81, 94], were performed in Japan. In two cases, HIT [72, 81] was also present and in three cases the PVT was accompanied by hepatic vein thrombosis (HVT, Budd-Chiari syndrome) [72, 81, 87]. Because treatment and prevention of PVT is an off label indication for danaparoid the dosing regimen used in Japan was that approved for DIC treatment, i.e. 1250–2500 U/day as 1 or 2 i.v. bolus injections (or short infusions) respectively. For most patients the higher dose 1250 U b.d., i.v. was chosen. In the three non-Japanese single case reports [72, 81, 91] the danaparoid regimen was 'therapeutic' (i.e. >2250 U/day) to treat HIT resulting from initial use of a heparin for the PVT and/or the HVT. In one of these patients it was used safely up to and after orthotopic liver transplant and to anticoagulate the cell saver during surgery [81]. For the other HIT patient no precise dosing information is available and for the third non-Japanese patient [93], the dose was also not mentioned but it was administered with warfarin until the patient could be discharged on warfarin only. Danaparoid exposure lasted a median 14 days (range 4 days to 2 months). In addition, sporadic reports state its successful re-use when PVT recurred during long-term warfarin use [55, 59, 67, 70].

Fifteen reports showed that AT was used concomitantly with danaparoid in 180 patients and in 2 studies AT was used alone as a comparator in 93 patients. In some studies comparing danaparoid alone with danaparoid + AT the AT was only used in patients presenting with plasma levels below 60%. The AT regimen was usually 1500 U daily for 3 days, but in one comparative study [56] and one case report [88] it was administered for 5 days. Administration of AT was often dependent upon the patient's AT status but in two studies danaparoid alone was compared with danaparoid + AT.

4.1.3 Results

The efficacy of danaparoid treatment assessed as complete, ≥70%, 50%–70%, <50% recanalisation/no change or as a new/progressive thrombosis, are summarised in **Table 6**.

Danaparoid treatment was associated with complete recanalisation in 46% of the patients and clinically significant thrombosis management in 72.6% (i.e. ≥70% PVT resolution) of the patients (although some investigators considered >50% reduction as clinically significant). An ineffective outcome was recorded in 10.7% of the patients including one with progression of thrombosis. Two studies assessed vessel volume reduction as a measure of recanalisation. One [61], involving 41 patients treated with danaparoid only, expressed the result as the mean reduction of 55.1% ± 40.2% at

Treatment	*n*	Outcome of PVT treatment				
		Degree of PVT resolution				New/progression of thrombus
		Complete	≥70%	50%–70%	<50%/nc	
Danaparoid only all studies	270	94	124	34	12	6
		34.8%	45.9%	12.6%	4.4%	2.2%
Danaparoid + AT all studies	87	24	34	9	20	0
		27.6%	39.1%	10.3%	23.0%	
All danaparoid	370	173	97	61	38	1 0.3%
		46.8%	26.2%	16.5%	10.3%	
AT only	24	11/24	nd	nd	nd	nd
		45.8%				

nc = no change, AT = antithrombin, nd = no data.

Table 6.
Pooled outcomes of PVT treatment.

2 weeks, the other [66], involving 55 patients also treated with danaparoid only, found a reduction from median 3.43 cm^3 to 1.42 cm^3, also at 2 weeks. Incidental presenting thromboses were: SSST and ovarian vein in one patient and two PEs, all resolved during danaparoid treatment, but only one of the three concomitant hepatic vein thromboses responded favourably to danaparoid. In all reports providing data on coagulation markers D-dimer, TAT and fibrinogen the plasma levels normalised by 2 weeks. All platelet counts (including the two patients with HIT) also increased to normal except for one patient, but no reason was given. In addition, plasma AT levels, whether above 60% before danaparoid treatment initiation or supplemented with injected AT, did not deteriorate during danaparoid use. The only study with a group of non-anticoagulated controls showed.

Three bleeding events (0.8%) developed, one each in three patients, during danaparoid treatment initiation: two from varices (one following endoscopic ligation), and one peritoneal haemorrhage. Danaparoid was restarted in one. No problem was recorded during the transition from danaparoid to warfarin.

No patient death was reported within 3 months of stopping danaparoid treatment. Other adverse events reported were the development of ascites in two patients (one with diarrhoea) and one case of thrombocytopenia that was not considered serious but no other details were provided. Despite one investigator [56] calculating that warfarin doubled the time of PVT recurrence from 1 to 2 years, eight others [55–59, 61, 66, 67] reported that follow-up treatment with warfarin failed to maintain PVT reductions achieved when danaparoid was discontinued.

4.1.4 Indirect comparison of danaparoid with other anticoagulants

Due to the lack of adequate non danaparoid and or AT controls an indirect comparison of pooled PVT treatment outcomes with various other drug treatment strategies has been made in **Table 7**. These data [95–107], however, lack consistency in describing PVT treatment outcomes. Hence it was necessary to express the results as complete and ≥50%. Despite this restriction it appears that clinically relevant PVT resolution, i.e. complete or ≥70% recanalisation, occurred in 73% of danaparoid treated patients compared with <42% for no treatment, <62% for sulodexide and <67% for the LMWH. It is not possible to calculate for warfarin but it is also in likely to be in the region of 70%. Thus the efficacy of danaparoid is at least as good as warfarin and the LMWH. However the frequencies of no change or progression of the PVT and bleeding was much lower with danaparoid.

Comparison with non-danaparoid controls other than AT is confounded by: the fact that only two small studies [54, 58] used such controls. One study tested danaparoid prophylaxis and found that no PVTs in the 11 danaparoid treated patients but 2 in the 32 patients receiving AT only. The two PVTs and seven from a prior 'testing' cohort in this study were successfully treated with danaparoid. In a study of cirrhosis related PVT [54] danaparoid successfully managed all eight PVTs in its treatment group but of the seven UFH + Urokinase controls only five (71.4%) responded favourably and the two non-responders died of liver failure within 3 months of treatment. While there is little evidence from non-danaparoid controls in the danaparoid studies there is evidence based on the use of the heparins and VKA that anticoagulation increases the chance of recanalisation of PVT. However if recurrences are to be prevented it is also necessary to follow-up with long term outpatient anticoagulation. This has largely been left to the VKAs but more recently the oral direct oral anticoagulants (DOACs) have also become available.

Antithrombotic treatment	*n*	Outcome of PVT treatment[1]					Bleeding events
		Extent of PVT resolution				New or TE extension	
		Complete	≥70%	50%–70%	<50% or nc		
LMWHs[2]	298	86	97		67	22	26
		31.6%	35.7%[3]		24.6%	8.1%	9.6%
Warfarin	121		82 83.7%		12	4	23
					12.2%	4.1%	23.5%
Sulodexide	32	5	8		8	0	11
		23.8%	38.1%		38.1%		52.4%
None	209	7	103		45	49	5
		2.6%	38.6%		20.3%[4]	22.1%[4]	1.9%
Danaparoid	357	118	158	43	32	6	3
		33.1%	44.3%	12.0%	9.0%	1.7%	0.8%

nc = no change, TE = thrombi, LMWHs = low molecular weight heparins.
[1]in many reports PVT resolution expressed only as complete or ≥50%.
[2]LMWH unspecified, enoxaparin and nadroparin.
[3]only >50% resolution data for all studies.
[4]in one study of 20 patients data for <50% resolution and recurrence were combined (12 = 60.0%) hence the study has been excluded from the calculation.

Table 7.
Comparison of pooled published non-danaparoid PVT outcomes with pooled danaparoid outcomes.

5. Danaparoid prophylaxis of post-transplant thrombotic disorders

The diagnosis of SOS is usually based on the Baltimore or Seattle criteria, and not every publication—especially single case reports or meeting abstracts, reveals which was used. The main difference between these two diagnostic guidelines is the inclusion of hyperbilirubinemia in the former. This seemingly small difference can result in great differences in important outcome events such as TRM, OS and MOD/MOF frequencies [108] when applied within the same population cohort. The European Society for Blood and Marrow Transplantation (EBMT) has attempted to rationalise this by applying the two sets of criteria to early and late SOS since hyperbilirubinemia is often absent in late SOS but a grey area remains and the change has yet to be clinically validated. Such validation is necessary since it appears to have a great influence on disease progression and the outcomes of specific treatment modalities.

5.1 Population exposure

Danaparoid has been evaluated in at least 524 patients for the prevention of SOS and/or TA-TMA after HSCT. All eight reports [108–115] come from Japan. Malignancies, particularly haematogenous cancers, formed about 80% of the reasons for HSCT. The non-malignant reasons were mainly aplastic anaemia, adrenoleukodystrophy and mucopolysaccharidoses. The subjects presented with a wide spectrum of underlying clinical disorders and had followed a course of chemotherapy (the conditioning regimen) or radiotherapy. In addition they had or were still receiving prophylaxis against GvHD and a cocktail of prophylactic medication to prevent BMT rejection and infection. Many of these drugs cause SOS or TA-TMA because of their hepato- and renal toxicity.

Japanese investigators have compared danaparoid use in both indications with standard prophylaxis using AT and/or ursodeoxycholic acid (UDCA) with or without antithrombotic co-medication. Defibrotide (DF) the standard therapy for SOS/TA-TMA treatment is also increasingly used for their prevention but there has not been a direct comparison with danaparoid.

The 197 patients in 2 comparative studies were adults [108] or mostly adults (median age 48 years, range 16–70 years) [109], as was one of the single cases reported [115]. The remaining studies and case reports of 326 patients were performed exclusively or mostly in children (age range < 1–18 years). In the only two studies with data males appeared to predominate (64.2%).

5.2 Study

The dosing regimens for danaparoid (provided in all but one case series and a single case report), dalteparin and UDCA in adults and children in the remaining reports are shown in **Table 8**. For danaparoid the adult regimen 2500 U/day follows that approved for DIC treatment in Japan and is close to the lower limit of the recommended dosing range for thrombosis treatment. This has been adapted for use in children and the 60–70 U/Kg/day is similar to that used for paediatric (V)TE treatment [116]. However this is equivalent to 4200–4900 U/day for a 70 kg adult, twice the dosing intensity received by adults for SOS/TA-TMA prevention.

5.3 Results

Many studies concentrated on SOS without mention of TMA, hence it is not known if TA-TMA was absent or not considered. The efficacy outcomes of these prophylactic studies with danaparoid were usually mainly expressed as outcome survival (OS) and treatment related mortality (TRM). All efficacy and bleeding outcomes are summarised in **Table 9**.

SOS/TA-TMA prophylaxis regimen	Dosing regimens of danaparoid and active controls used for SOS/TA-TMA prophylaxis[1]			
	Adults		Children	
	n	Dosing regimen	*n*	Dosing regimen
Danaparoid used alone	164	1250 U b.d., i.v.	0	—
Danaparoid (+ UDCA)	33	1250 U o.d.,i.v.	223	30 U/kg b.d.,i.v.
Dalteparin used alone	59	3000 IU/day as i.v. infusion	0	—
Dalteparin (+ UDCA)	52	2500–3500 IU/day	96	70 IU/Kg/day
UDCA used alone	195	600 mg/day	0	—
UDCA + antithrombotic	85	300–600 mg/day	210	10 mg/kg/day

b.d. twice daily, o.d. once daily, i.v. = intravenous, UDCA = ursodeoxycholic acid.
[1]for 1 adult and 103 children no dosing regimen is available.

Table 8.
Dosing regimens used for danaparoid and controls for SOS/TA-TMA prophylaxis.

Antithrombotic and/or UDCA	*n*	SOS	TA-TMA	TRM	OS	GvHD	MB
Danaparoid only	255	23/255	11/255	14/255	191/255	51/164	4/164
		9.0%	4.3%	5.5%	74.9%	31.1%³	2.4%
Danaparoid + UDCA	268	24/202	nd	2/114	188/235	5/77	6/211
		11.9%		1.8%	80.0%	6.5%⁴	2.8%
Dalteparin only	59	13/59	nd	12/59	29/59	24/59	6/59
		22.0%		20.3%	49.2%	40.7%³	10.2%
Dalteparin + UDCA	148	22/148	nd	17/86	56/96	13/86	4/47
		14.9%		19.8%	58.3%	15.1%⁴	8.5%
UDCA only	195	28/195	nd	16/195	nd	nd	10/195
		14.4%		8.2%			5.1%

Dan = danaparoid, (LMW)H = low and unfractionated heparins, MB = major bleeding, nd = no or unclear data, OS = outcome survival, SOS = sinusoidal obstruction syndrome, TA-TMA transplant associated thrombotic microangiopathy, TRM = treatment related mortality, UDCA = urso-deoxycholic acid.
[1]early and late refer only to TA-TMA <2 weeks or ≥ 4 weeks respectively, and to TRM ≤3 months or 2–5 years respectively, according to the publications with data on either or both.
[2]nd = no data or in some cases insufficient clarity of data (mortality rate compared in terms of p values or cumulative frequency charts).
[3]total is for only acute GvHD (grade II–IV) at 3 months.
[4]total is for acute GvHD (grade II-IV) at 3 months plus chronic GvHD.

Table 9.
Pooled treatment outcomes of SOS/TA-TMA prevention in danaparoid studies.

Not all parameters were addressed in each of the seven studies therefore % frequency calculations have been corrected by the available data. This indirect comparison suggests that danaparoid reduces SOS/TA-TMA frequency in patients undergoing HSCT at least as well as a LMWH and UDCA with a lower frequency of bleeding at the dosing regimen used. More importantly it appears that danaparoid ± UDCA reduced TRM. Unfortunately the study with a UDCA treatment only control [99] did not provide information on TRM or OS development and for an unexplained reason halved the dose of danaparoid to 1250 U o.d.

5.4 Adverse events

The frequency of major bleeding events was lowest in patients receiving danaparoid. The development of GvHD was only mentioned in two study reports with grossly disparate results (see **Table 9**) between anticoagulant alone or combined with UDCA. One dalteparin treated subject developed HIT [105] but there is no record of how this was treated. Two danaparoid treated patients developed DIC. Of the 16 patients undergoing allogenic SCT for Adrenoleukodystrophy [108] transient haemolytic anaemia (2), engraftment syndrome (9) and viral reactivation developed all of which improved with specific treatment or supportive care while danaparoid treatment continued.

Of the 5 specifically paediatric studies three [110, 111, 114] reported no post-BMT complications and two [112, 113] reported 27 patients (8.3%) with SOS, TA-TMA or DIC associated with sepsis or engraftment syndrome. All were successfully treated with recombinant thrombomodulin.

6. Other treatments for SOS/TA-TMA

Currently while several drugs for SOS prophylaxis are available there is no clear treatment to prevent TA-TMA.

6.1 The heparins

Despite some reports of successful prophylaxis with UFH and LMWHs a meta-analysis and systematic review of their use [117] found no significant reduction in risk of SOS. Safety also appeared to be an issue when used in patients with gastro-intestinal varices or thrombocytopenia or renal dysfunction, especially when they were combined with lipo-prostaglandin E1 or UDCA. Hence heparin is no longer recommended for SOS prophylaxis [20].

6.2 Ursodeoxycholic acid

UDCA, currently the most widely used drug for SOS prevention, is a natural bile acid that is capable of reducing the toxicity of its companion bile acids in cholestatic liver diseases. In inflammatory disorders it can 'attenuate the pro-inflammatory cytokine environment through decreased expression of TNF-α, interleukins 1 and 2, and interferon-γ, thereby minimising endothelial injury occurring in HSCT associated with the cytokine storm [117]. UDCA is safe and not only lowers the frequency of SOS but also of TRM and appears to have a small effect in reducing the development

Antithrombotic and/or UDCA	***n***	**SOS**	**TRM**	**OS**	**GvHD**	**MB**
Danaparoid only						
All	255	9.0%	5.5%	74.9%	31.1%	2.4%
Adults	164	10.4%	8.6%	65.2%	31.1%	3.7%
Children	91	6.8%	0.0%	92.3%	nd	0.0%
Danaparoid + UDCA						
All	268	11.9%	nd	74.6%	6.5%	2.8%
Adults	33	15.2%	nd	65.2%	nd	3.0%
Children	235	4.1%	1.8%	80.0%	9.1%	1.5%
UDCA only	1441	14.4%	8.2%	nd	nd	5.1%
DF 'only'[5]	1371	4.9%	19.0%	72.3%	22.2%	22%
DF + UDCA[6]	56	1.9%	1.9%	nd	nd	nd

Dan = danaparoid, DF = defibrotide, GvHD = graft v host disease, (LMW)H = low and unfractionated heparins, MB = major bleeding, nd = no or unclear data, OS = outcome survival, SOS = sinusoidal obstruction syndrome, TA-TMA transplant associated thrombotic microangiopathy, TRM = treatment related mortality, UDCA = urso-deoxycholic acid.
[1]*From* **Table 9**
[2]*From* **Table 9** *and additional data from non-danaparoid studies.*
[3]*Assessed at either D + 100 and/or 2–5 years after HSCT, OS was 100% for danaparoid + UDCA.*
[4]*Assessed at D + 100 after HSCT.*
[5]*From Refs. [119, 120]*
[6]*From Ref. [121]*

Table 10.
Pooled results of SOS prophylaxis studies.

of GvHD [118]. It is occasionally used in combination with UFH and LMWHs but there is little evidence that they improve its efficacy. Outcomes of UDCA use shown in **Table 10** are derived from several studies and reviews [117–120, 122].

6.3 Defibrotide

This oligodesoxyribonucleotide extracted from porcine intestinal mucosa has numerous antithrombotic, EC protective, fibrinolytic, anti-ischaemic and angiogenic activities. Its clear benefits for the treatment of SOS have led to approval by the FDA for this indication. More recently DF has been investigated for SOS prevention with mixed results [121, 123–127]. The inter-study variance may be due to the different dosing regimens used (including occasional co-medication with UDCA) and different intervals between diagnosis and DF treatment initiation. Greater success has been reported using initiating DF earlier [128] after SOS diagnosis or combining it with UDCA [129].

6.4 Results

The outcomes of non-danaparoid studies with UDCA and DF for the prevention of SOS (and where mentioned TA-TMA) are summarised and compared with danaparoid in **Table 10**. The data for danaparoid only and in combination with UDCA have been separated because of the apparent greater. Impact of comedication with UDCA on the frequencies of TRM and GvHD. For many studies it is unclear to what extent TA-TMA might have been present and therefore contributed to caused morbidity or death since it was mentioned. In addition not all parameters were assessed in all studies hence percentages are based only on the available data. The frequency of haemorrhages with DF in several studies [130, 131] has been as high as 22%, but in one study [130] was the same as the unspecified controls. So there remains some confusion regarding its safety.

Interestingly the danaparoid efficacy appears to be better in children than in adults, perhaps related to the use of a higher dosing intensity/kg body weight.

7. Discussion

7.1 Danaparoid dosing

Danaparoid dosed at 1250 U b.d., i.v. in adults and 30 U/kg body weight b.d., i.v. in children, appears to be effective and safe for the treatment of PVT or prevention of SOS and TA-TMA. Despite the relatively high danaparoid dosing intensity used in children there were no reports of bleeding complications in any of the studies and case reports supporting its safety in these vulnerable subjects.

Nevertheless, the intermittent dosing regimen based on DIC treatment used for both adults and children is unlikely to be optimal since it takes 2–3 days to reach steady state drug levels, produces post-injection peak levels of drug that could cause bleeding in high risk patients and pre-injection troughs with insufficient thrombosis protection. The antithrombotic action of danaparoid is shared between the 5% by weight HA-HS and the 80% by weight NA-HS subfractions of danaparoid with greatly different half-lives—25 and 7 h respectively. Hence by the time the next 12 hourly danaparoid injection is due there is much less of the NA-HS left in the circulation even at steady-state pharmacokinetics. This subfraction is largely responsible for the anti-inflammatory and immunosuppressive actions of danaparoid [34]. Hence for TE treatment PK modelling was used to determine a dosing regimen that provided circulating therapeutic danaparoid levels as quickly as possible and maintained the natural ratios of the HS-HS and NA-HS constituents continuously. The ideal regimen was found to be an i.v. loading dose of 2250 U (body weight adjusted—1250 U if <55 kg and 3000 U if >90 kg), followed by a continuous i.v. infusion of 400 U/h × 4 hours, followed by 300 U/h × 4 hours, followed by the maintenance infusion rate of 150–200 U/h for as long as considered necessary. This regimen immediately attains and maintains the target plasma anti-Xa activity range of 0.4 and 0.8 U/mL and outside Japan is approved for patients with thrombosis. This can be important for increasing the efficacy of danaparoid not only for PVT treatment but also for SOS/TA-TMA prevention since the inflammatory disturbances should respond better to the continuous presence of the NA-HS subfraction of danaparoid. If a bleeding risk is present then the daily danaparoid dosing intensity, can be lowered by reducing the loading dose size by 25%–50% and the maintenance infusion rate to 100–125 U/h.

7.2 PVT treatment

Due to differences in detail between guidelines for the management of PVT, some confusion remains surrounding attempts to evaluate and compare its alternative treatment strategies. Many clinical factors such as the distribution of Child-Pugh status, the cause of cirrhosis, the frequency of cirrhosis, varices or hepatocellular carcinoma, the distribution of PVST and grade of vessel obstruction at the time of antithrombotic initiation, the age of the thrombus, the presence of infection, the inclusion of different antithrombotics and their combination with either AT or UDCA. Furthermore there is a need to standardise what is considered a 'good clinical treatment outcome' for PVT. Is it complete recanalisation only [94], or ≥70% partial recanalisation [58] or is ≥50% [95] sufficient. What assessment criteria for an effect on PVT is best—reduction thrombus size, in vessel volume or in portal hypertension or a combination of these possible outcomes? For how long should study end-points be assigned to the original treatment drug—2 weeks, 4 weeks or 3 months after switching to an alternative long-term antithrombotic? Such details are crucial for adequate drug comparisons. Even age and gender distributions of studies are not usually considered in the choice of studies included in meta-analyses but can have a profound effect on the clinical responses to treatment. For these reasons I am not convinced of the value of treatment assessment meta-analyses that are more concerned with the mechanics of study design [5, 14] than many of the above clinical issues.

The pooled results of danaparoid treatment suggest that it possesses at least the same efficacy as AT and its performance does not seem to be enhanced by the addition of AT. Danaparoid appears to be safe even in patients with moderate to severe hepatic dysfunction and extensive varices. A Japan-wide survey performed in 2018 [132], revealed that 46% of the 539 patients included in the responses were treated with danaparoid alone or + AT. A comparison of the outcomes of the six most common treatment regimens i.e. heparin, warfarin, danaparoid, heparin + warfarin, danaparoid + antithrombin and no anticoagulant, showed that warfarin produced the highest complete PVT disappearance rate (about 50% compared with danaparoid at 30%). However, the rate of PVT disappearance plus reduction (not defined) was highest for danaparoid about 80% compared with just over 70% for warfarin. The rates of no change and PVT extension were both lowest for danaparoid at about 18% and 2%

respectively. Furthermore, PVT disappearance rates with danaparoid + AT while better than those of heparin were inferior to those achieved with danaparoid alone.

7.3 SOS/TA-TMA prevention

Apart from one study [108] there appears to be agreement on the prophylactic dosing regimens of danaparoid used for adults or children to prevent SOS/TMA. Children above 2 years appear to require almost double the dosing intensity used in adults to achieve the same plasma anti-Xa levels [116], but it does not appear to have compromised safety in terms of bleeding and side-effects.

The study [109] that did not use UDCA co-medication recorded a higher rate of acute GvHD (grades II–IV) for both danaparoid alone and dalteparin alone compared with the much lower rates recorded for both drugs when combined with UCDA in the other major comparative study [110]. Whether this reveals a true effect of UDCA or a centre/patient cohort treatment bias requires further investigation. Acute GvHD is a risk factor for TA-TMA, thus it is unfortunate that the investigators [109] comparing a low intensity danaparoid + UDCA with dalteparin + UDCA and UDCA alone, although detailing measures taken to prevent GvHD, did not refer to it again.

Two comparative studies concluded that danaparoid: 'reduces the incidence of transplant associated microangiopathies' in adults [105] or 'lowers TRM after stem-cell transplantation in children' [110] since in both studies danaparoid was superior to dalteparin with or without UDCA. Whether or not these results are due to the anti-thrombotic action of danaparoid alone or a combination with its anti-inflammatory effects has not been investigated. The latter is likely in view of the positive results of danaparoid use in HIT [133], sepsis [134], APS [135, 136] and paroxysmal nocturnal haemoglobinuria [137].

7.4 HIT development

Although one patient exposed to danaparoid developed thrombocytopenia it was not reported to be due to HIT. However, of 214 control patients receiving UFH or a LMWH in the danaparoid studies a case of HIT was recorded [109].

7.5 Alternative therapies

Long term antithrombotic treatment appears to be crucial for preventing PVT recurrences and the VKAs have until recently been the method of choice. However, despite one investigator [56] calculating that warfarin doubled the time of PVT recurrence from 1 to 2 years, eight others [55–59, 61, 62, 67] reported that follow-up treatment with warfarin after initial danaparoid failed to maintain PVT reductions achieved when danaparoid was discontinued. A comparison of warfarin v edoxaban following danaparoid PVT reduction showed that only edoxaban maintained or reduced the already achieved vessel volume reduction.

Whether any pharmaceutical prophylaxis for SOS/TATMA is effective remains controversial, but it appears possible with current therapy options and UDCA is now recommended by the EBMT Handbook and the British Committee for Standards in Haematology/British Society for Blood and Marrow Transplantation guidelines. It is unclear if UDCA improves the efficacy of danaparoid but it appears to improve the safety of DF in patients with a high risk of developing SOS. It is also unclear who should receive prophylaxis and which treatment is most likely to offer the best risk–benefit ratio so it is interesting that danaparoid is especially effective in reducing both SOS and TRM in children and increases their OS.

DF appears to be efficacious in preventing SOS but at the expense of a high bleeding rate (perhaps related to its pro-fibrinolytic activity). A large prospective Phase III controlled trial of DF v best management without DF was discontinued in 2018. The manufacturers report of the interim analysis of that study concluded 'it would be highly unlikely to reach statistical significance for the primary end-point of SOS survival at Day +30 post HSCT in the final analysis if the study were to complete enrolment' [138]. So that there remains confusion around the evidence for DFG suitability for SOS prophylaxis. Danaparoid however, appears to be safe even when compared with UDCA.

7.6 Cost calculations

It is difficult to generalise about the cost effectiveness of different pharmacological strategies for SOS prevention due to the unclear duration of drug administration and inter-country differences in basic drug and hospitalisation costs. In Europe the current price of 10 × 750 U ampoules of danaparoid sodium varies between € 975 and € 1250 (price discounting not considered), having been much less when originally approved for DVT prophylaxis. Thus per patient treatment of PVT at 3 A/day for 2 weeks could cost about € 5250. For SOS/TA-TMA prophylaxis danaparoid administration at 3–4 A/day for the median 2 months treatment duration would cost between € 17,500 and € 30,000. This assumes long term follow-up treatment with a VKA or DOAC to prevent recurrence of the PVT. For DF dosed at 25 mg/kg/day divided into 4 doses the drug cost is about the same as danaparoid. DF is known to reduce hospital stay but this effect is somewhat offset by the fact that unlike danaparoid many patients do not complete their treatment due to adverse events, particularly bleeding and these events incur the costs of additional investigations and treatment. One single centre study [139] found an SOS incidence of 7.4% and a TRM of 19%. Their cost effectiveness analysis led to the conclusion that 'prophylactic DF for children at risk of SOS was not cost-effective with respect to TRM and length of hospital stay'. By contrast the UDCA cost per patient (in 2013) was about € 400 for 2 months treatment [140]. UDCA can be a lifelong treatment but and its cost price may have risen since then. Which is the most cost-effective for the management of SOS/TA-TMA hinges on the desired outcome—mere prevention or reducing TRM and increasing OS.

8. Conclusions

Problems associated with study design, diagnostic criteria, end-point choice and evaluation, and use of single or several pharmacological agent, make it difficult to evaluate and compare the outcomes of different drug trials in hepatic thrombotic disorders.

Despite the absence of studies against placebo/no treatment to establish absolute efficacy, comparative studies versus a LMWH suggest that danaparoid is effective and safe for the treatment of PVT and not only prevents SOS and TA-TMA but reduces TRM and increases OS after HSCT. It is unclear if the efficacy of danaparoid is improved with the addition of AT or UDCA.

Danaparoid has a high cost of treatment but a cost-efficacy analysis has not been performed. Its safety, particularly the low haemorrhagic risk, may offset some of these costs.

Given the potentially fatal outcomes of hepatic thrombotic disorders, the ease of administration of danaparoid, its apparent efficacy and safety in patients with a high bleeding risk, danaparoid merits further investigation in the management of hepatic thrombotic disorders. However the dose of danaparoid needs to be optimised.

There remains a great need for sufficiently powered, double-blind, randomised controlled trials, with well defined end-points relevant for clinical practise, to evaluate the short and long-term effects of currently available antithrombotics used in the management of hepatic thrombotic disorders.

Conflict of interest

The author declares no conflict of interest.

Author details

Harry N. Magnani
Oss, The Netherlands

*Address all correspondence to: harry.magnani@hetnet.nl

References

[1] Lautt WW, Greenway CV. Conceptual review of the hepatic vascular bed. Hepatology. 1987;7:952

[2] Myers JD, Hickam JB. An estimation of the hepatic blood flow and splanchnic oxygen consumption in heart failure. The Journal of Clinical Investigation. 1948;**27**:620

[3] Lisman T, Hernandez-Gea V, Magnusson M, Roberts L, Stanworth S, Thachill J, et al. The concept of rebalanced haemostasis in patients with liver disease: Communication from the ISTH SSC working group on haemostatic management of patients with liver disease. Journal of Thrombosis and Haemostasis. 2021;**19**:1116-1122

[4] Rattner DW, Ellman L, Warshaw AL. Portal vein thrombosis after elective splenectomy. An underappreciated, potentially lethal syndrome. Archives of Surgery. 1993;**128**:565-570

[5] Zhang N, Yao Y, Xue W, Wu S. Early prophylactic anticoagulation for portal venous system thrombosis after splenectomy: A systematic review and meta-analysis. Biomedical Reports. 2016;**5**:483-490

[6] Plessier A, Darwish-Murad S, Hernandez-Guerra M, Consigny Y, Fabris F, Trebicka I, et al. European network for vascular disorders of the liver (EN-VIE). Acute portal vein thrombosis unrelated to cirrhosis: A prospective multicenter follow-up study. Hepatology. 2010;**51**(1):210-218. DOI: 10.1002/hep.23259

[7] Rokkam VRP, Sridharan GK, Vegunta R, Boregowda U, Moha BP. Clostridium difficile and COVID-19: Novel risk factors for acute portal vein thrombosis. Case Reports in Vascular Medicine. 2021;**2021**:883263. DOI: 10.1155/2021/8832638

[8] Franco-Moreno A, Piniella-Ruiz E, Montoya-Adarraga J, Ballano-Franco C, Alvarez-Miguel F, Peinado-Martinez C, et al. Portal vein thrombosis in a patient with COVID-19. Thrombosis Research. 2020;**194**:150-152

[9] Porres-Aguilar M, Lazo-Langner A, Panduro A, Uribe M. COVID-19 vaccine -induced immune thrombotic thrombocytopenia: An emerging cause of splanchnic vein thrombosis. Annals of Hepatology. 2021;**23**:100356

[10] Manzano-Robleda MC, Barranco-Fragoso B, Uribe M, Méndez-Sánchez N. Portal vein thrombosis: What is new? Annals of Hepatology. 2015;**14**(1):20-27. DOI: 10.1016/S1665-2681(19)30797-5

[11] Mantaka A, Augoustaki A, Kouroumalis EA, Samonakis DN. Portal vein thrombosis in cirrhosis: Diagnosis, natural history, and therapeutic challenges. Annals of Gastroenterology. 2018;**31**(3):315-329. DOI: 10.20524/aog.2018.0245

[12] Intagliata NM, Ferriera CM, Caldwell SH. Anticoagulation for portal vein thrombosis. Clinical Liver Disease. 2016;**7**(6):126-130

[13] Wu M, Schuster M, Tadros M. Update on management of portal vein thrombosis and the role of novel anticoagulants. Journal of Clinical and Translational Hepatology. 2019;**7**(2):152-164

[14] Qi X, De Stefano V, Li H, Dai J, Guo X, Fan D. Anticoagulation for the treatment of portal vein thrombosis in

liver cirrhosis: A systemic review and meta-analysis of observational studies. European Journal of Internal Medicine. 2015;**26**:23-29

[15] Bonifazi F, Barbato F, Favaioli F, Sessa M, Difrancesco I, Arpinati N, et al. Diagnosis and treatment of VOD/SOS after hematopoietic stem cell transplantation. Frontiers in Immunology. 2020;**11**:489. DOI: 10.3389/fimmu.2020.00489

[16] Jodelle S, Medvedovic M, Leubbering N, Chen J, Dandoy CE, Laskin BL, et al. Interferon-complement loop in transplant associated thrombotic microangiopathy. Blood Advances. 2020;**4**(6):1166-1177

[17] Mezo B, Horvath O, Sinkovits G, Veszeli N, Krivan G, Prohaszka Z. Vailidation of early increase activation marker cC5b-9 as a predictive biomarker for the development of thrombotic microangiopathy after stem cell transplantation. Frontiers in Medicine. 2020;**7**:1-10. Article: 569291. DOI: 10.3389/fmed.2020.569291

[18] Gavriilaki E, Ho VT, Schwaeble W, Dudler T, Daha M, Fujita T, et al. Role of the lectin pathway of complement in hematopoietic stem-cell transplantation-associated endothelial injury and thrombotic microangiopathy. Experimental Hematology & Oncology. 2021;**10**(57). DOI: 10.1186/s40164-021-00249-8

[19] Vion A-C, Rautou P-E, Durand F, Boulanger C, Valla D. Interplay of inflammation and endothelial dysfunction in bone marrow transplantation: Focus on hepatic veno-occlusive disease. Seminars in Thrombosis and Hemostasis. 2015;**41**:629-643. DOI: 10.1055/s-0035-1556728

[20] Arai Y, Yamashita K, Mizugishi K, Watanabe T, Sakamoto S, Kitano T, et al. Serum neutrophil extracellular trap levels predict thrombotic microangiopathy after allogeneic stem cell transplantation. Biology of Blood and Marrow Transplantation. 2013;**19**(12):1683-1689

[21] Carreras E, on behalf of the Barcelona Endothelium Team (BET). Vascular endothelial syndromes after HSCT. Bone Marrow Transplantation. 2020;**2020**(55):1885-1887

[22] Pagliuca S, Michonneau D, Sicre de Fnotbrune S, Sutra del Galy A, Xhaard A, Robin M, et al. Allogenic-reactivity mediated endothelial complications after HSCT: A plea for consensual definitions. Blood Advances. 2019;**3**:2424-2435

[23] Bucalossi A, Toraldo F, Lenoci M, Castangnini C, Artuso R, Renieri A, et al. Is complement alternative pathway dysregulation involved in veno-occlusive disease of the liver? Biology of Blood and Marrow Transplantation. 2010;**16**:1749-1750

[24] Hildebrandt GC, Chao N. Endothelial cell function and endothelial-related disorders following haematopoietic cell transplantation. British Journal of Haematology. 2020;**190**:508-519. DOI: 10.1111/bjh.16621

[25] Dalle JH, Giralt SA. Hepatic veno-occlusive disease after hematopoietic stem-cell transplantation: Risk factors and stratification, prophylaxis and treatment. Biology of Blood and Marrow Transplantation. 2016;**22**:400-409. DOI: 10.1016/j.bbmt.2015.09.024

[26] Ye Y, Zheng W, Wang J, Hu Y, Luo Y, Tan Y, et al. Risk and prognostic factors for transplantation associated thrombotic microangiopathy in allogeneic haematopoietic stem cell transplantation: A nested case control study. Journal of Hematology & Oncology. 2016;**35**(4):

821-827. Published on-line. DOI: 10.1002/hon.2310

[27] Elfeky R, Lucchini G, Lum SH, et al. New insights into risk factor for transplant-associated thrombotic microangiopathy (TA-TMA) in paediatric HSCT. J Blood Adv. 2020;**4**(11):2418-2429

[28] Dvorak CC, Higham C, Shimano KA. Transplant associated thrombotic microangiopathy in pediatric hematopoietic cell transplant recipients: A practical approach to diagnosis and management. Frontiers in Pediatrics. 2019;7:133. DOI: 10.3389/fped.2019.00133

[29] Young JA, Pallas CR, Knovich MA. Transplant associated thrombotic microangiopathy: Theoretical considerations and a practical approach to an unrefined diagnosis. Bone Marrow Transplantation. 2021;**56**:1805-1817. DOI: 10.1038/s41409-021-01283-i0

[30] Kavanagh D, Richards A, Atkinson J. Complement regulatory genes and hemolytic-uremic syndromes. Annual Review of Medicine. 2008;**59**:293-309

[31] Stanford KI, Wang L, Castagnola J, Song D, Bishop JR, Brown JR, et al. Journal of Biological Chemistry. 2010;**285**(1):286-294

[32] Farrugia BL, Lord MS, Melrose J, Whitelock JM. The role of heparan sulphate in inflammation, and the development of biomimetics as anti-inflammatory strategies. Journal of Histochemistry and Cytochemistry. 2018;**66**:321-328. DOI: 10.1369/0022155417740881

[33] Chong BH, Burgess J, Ismail F. The clinical usefulness of the platelet aggregation test for the diagnosis of heparin-induced thrombocytopenia. Thrombosis and Haemostasis. 1993;**69**:344-350

[34] Greinacher A, Michels I, Muller-Eckhardt C. Heparin-associated thrombocytopenia: The antibody is not heparin specific. Thrombosis and Haemostasis. 1992;**67**:545-549

[35] Krauel K, Furll B, Warkentin TE, Weitschies W, Kohlmann T, Sheppard JI, et al. Heparin-induced thrombocytopenia: Therapeutic concentrations of danaparoid unlike fondaparinux and direct thrombin inhibitors inhibit formation of platelet factor 4-heparin complexes. Journal of Thrombosis and Haemostasis. 2008;**6**:2160-2167

[36] Risi G. Characterization PF4-heparin complexes by photon correlation spectroscopy and zeta potential. Report from Istituto di Recherche Chimiche e Biochimiche 'G. Ronzoni', Milan Italy. 2016

[37] Fujishima Y, Yokota K, Sukamoto T. The effect of danaparoid sodium (danaparoid) on endotoxin-induced experimental disseminated intravascular coagulation (DIC) in rats. Thrombosis Research. 1998;**91**:221-227

[38] Iba T, Kidokoro A, Fukunaga M, Nagakari K, Suda M, Yoshikawa S, et al. Antithrombin ameliorates endotoxin-induced organ dysfunction more efficiently when combined with danaparoid sodium than with infractionated heparin. Intensive Care Medicine. 2005;**31**:1101-1108

[39] Mizutani A, Mizutani S, Noguchi T, Murakami K, Saito H, Enkhbaatar P, et al. Danaparoid reduces combined burn and smoke inhalation-induced acute lung injury in mice by activation of capsaicin-sensitive sensory neurons. Critical Care Medicine. 2005;**33**(12):A8 Abstract 32

[40] Mizutani A, Mizutani S, Noguchi T, Kudo K, Hidaka S, Takatani J, et al.

Danaparoid reduces ischaemia/reperfusion-induced acute renal injury in rats by activation of capsaicin-sensitive sensory neurons. Critical Care Medicine. 2005;**33**(12 Suppl):A147 Poster150-T

[41] Iba T, Miyasho T. Danaparoid sodium attenuates the increase in inflammatory cytokines and preserves organ function in endotoxaemic rats. Critical Care. 2008;**12**(4) e-pub

[42] Harada N, Okajima K, Kohmura H, Uchiba M, Tomita T. Danaparoid sodium reduces ischaemia/reperfusion-induced liver injury in rats by attenuating inflammatory responses. Thrombosis and Haemostasis. 2007;**91**:81-87

[43] Hagiwara S, Iwasaka H, Hidaki S, Noguchi T. Danaparoid sodium inhibits systemic inflammation and prevents endotoxin-induced acute lung injury in rats. Critical Care. 2008;**12**(2):R43. DOI: 10.1186/cc6851. [Epub Apr 2, 2008]. PMID: 18380908; PMCID: PMC2447588

[44] Shimosawa M, Sakamoto K, Kamikado K, Otsuka H, Liu N, Kitamura H, et al. Lipopolysaccharide-triggered aggravation of acute mesangio-proliferative glomerulonephritis through activation of coagulation in a high IgA strain of ddY mice. Experimental Nephrology. 2009;**112**(4):e81-e91

[45] Hagiwara S, Iwasaka H, Shingu C, Matsumoto S, Uchida T, Nishida T, et al. Danaparoid sodium attenuates the effects of heat stroke. Journal of Surgical Research. 2011;**171**:762-768

[46] Hino H, Miura A, Shin M, Kon W, Tateda T. Administration of AT in conjunction with danaparoid improves nerve conduction in the peripheral nerves of rats administered with LPS over a period of 48 hours. Anesthesia and Analgesia. 2011;**112** Abstract S-97

[47] Lu X, Zhao L, Xu Y-H. Low molecular weight heparin prevents CLP-induced acute lung injury in rats by anti-inflammatory coagulation. Bosnian Journal of Basic Medical Sciences. 2013;**13**(1):50-56

[48] Wang X, Tanino Y, Nikaido T, Kikuchi M, Sato Y, Fukuhara M, et al. Danaparoid attenuates bleomycin-induced pulmonary fibrosis in mice. American Journal of Respiratory and Critical Care Medicine. 2016;**193**:A4156

[49] Bargues L, Foissard B, Jault P, Samson T, Carsin H. Heparin-induced thrombocytopenia: Report of four cases in severely burned patients. Annales Françaises d'Anesthèsie et de Rèanimation. 2006;**25**(11-12):1135-1139

[50] Sobczak AIS, Pitt SJ, Stewart AJ. Glycosaminoglycan neutralization in coagulation control. Arteriosclerosis, Thrombosis, and Vascular Biology. 2018;**38**(6):1258-1270. DOI: 10.1161/ATVBAHA.118.311102

[51] Weitz JI. Heparan sulfate: Antithrombotic or not? Journal of Clinical Investigation. 2003;**111**:952-954. DOI: 10.1172/JCI200318234

[52] Schriver Z. Heparin and heparan sulphate: Analysing structure and microheterogeneity. Handbook of Experimental Pharmacology. 2012;**207**:159-176. DOI: 10.1007/978-3-642-23056-1_8

[53] Griffin KL, Fischer BM, Kummarapurugu AB, Zheng S, Kennedy TP, Rao NV, et al. 2-O, 3-desulphated heparin inhibits neutrophil elastase-induced HMGB-1 secretion and airway inflammation. American Journal of Respiratory Cell and Molecular Biology. 2014;**50**(1):684-689

[54] Haga H, Nishina T, Mizuno K, Katsumi T, Okumoto K, Saito T, et al. The efficacy of danaparoid sodium on portal thrombosis in patients with hepatic cirrhosis. Hepatology International. 2016;**10**(1 Suppl. 1):S373-S374

[55] Hayashi T, Takatori H, Horii R, Nio K, Tershima T, Lida N, et al. Danaparoid based anticoagulation therapy for portal vein thrombosis in cirrhotic patients. BMC Gastroenterology. 2019;**19**:217

[56] Takatori H, Hayashi T, Sunagozaka H, Arai K, Kitamura K, Kagaya T, et al. Danaparoid sodium monotherapy for portal vein thrombosis in cirrhotic patients is as effective as combination therapy with antithrombin III. Hepatology. 2013;**54**(Suppl. 4):894A

[57] Yamada R, Sakamori R, Kodama T, Shigekawa M, Hikita H, Tatsumi T, et al. The efficacy of anticoagulation treatment for portal vein thrombosis. Hepatology. 2018;**68**(Suppl. 1):1146A Poster 2030

[58] Kawanaka H, Akahoshi T, Ito S, Iguchi T, Harimoto N, Uchiyama H, Yoshizumi T, Shirabe K, Takenaka K, Maehara. Optimizing risk stratification in portal vein thrombosis after splenectomy and its primary prophylaxis with antithrombin III concentrates and danaparoid sodium in liver cirrhosis and portal hypertension. Journal of the American College of Surgeons 2014;**219**(5):865-874

[59] Fujiyama S, Saitoh S, Kawamura Y, Sezaki H, Hosaka T, Akuta N, et al. Portal vein thrombosis in liver cirrhosis. BMC Gastroenterology. 2017;**17**:112-120

[60] Imamura J, Osawa Y, Kimura K. The effectiveness of danaparoid sodium for portal vein thrombosis. Hepatology International. 2016;**10**(1 Suppl. 1):S89

[61] Kawamura E, Enomoto M, Kotani K, Motoyama H, Kozuka R, Hagihara A, et al. Danaparoid sodium thrombolytic therapy followed by warfarin in cirrhotic portal venous thrombosis. Hepatology International. 2016;**10**(1 Suppl. 1):S374

[62] Ohtake T, Tsuji K, Kawanishi T, Machida T, Takagi H, Mezawa S, et al. A multicentre survey of the efficacy and safety of danaparoid sodium treatment for portal vein thrombosis. Hepatology. 2014;**60**(4 Suppl. 1):399A Abstract 402

[63] Shudo R, Yazaki Y, Honda M, Sugawara K, Maeda S, Yoshizaki H, et al. Anticoagulation therapy with danaparoid sodium for portal vein thrombosis. American Journal of Gastroenterology. 2007;**102**:S215-S248 Abstract 336

[64] Ando S, Imai Y, Fichigami A, Nakazawa M, Mochida S. Usefulness of balloon-occluded retrograde transverse obliteration for the treatment of portal vein thrombosis in patients with liver cirrhosis. Journal of Gastroenterology and Hepatology. 2014;**29**(Suppl. 3):180 P368

[65] Inao M, Hirahara K, Sugawara K, Nakayama N, Imai Y, Mochida S. Usefulness of balloon occluded retrograde obliteration (B-RTO) as a consolidation procedure after anticoagulation therapy in cirrhotic patients with portal vein thrombosis. Hepatology. 2015;**62**(Suppl. 1):935A

[66] Nagaoki Y, Aikata H, Daijyo K, Teraoka Y, Shinohara F, Nakamura Y, et al. Efficacy and safety of edoxaban for treatment of portal vein thrombosis following danaparoid sodium in patients with liver cirrhosis. Hepatology Research. 2018;**48**(1):51-58. DOI: 10.1111/hepr.12895

[67] Fukuda W, Mori T, Mitsumoto Y, Hurose R, Naito T, Minami R, et al. A case of portal vein thrombosis successfully treated with danaparoid

sodium. Jpn J Publ Health. 2010;**16**: 193-198

[68] Hayashi M, Sugaya T, Fujita M, Nakamura J, Imaizumi H, Abe K, et al. Sigmoid colon varices due to massive thrombosis of a noncirrhotic extrahepatic portosystemic shunt. Internal Medicine. 2020. DOI: 10.2169/international medicine.4025-20

[69] Imaoka K, Fukuda S, Tazawa H, Fukuhara S, Hirata Y, Fujisaki S, et al. A rare case of pyelophlebitis as a complication of cholecystocolonic fistula. Surgical Case Reports. Nov 4, 2018;**2018**. Article: 3931674. DOI: 10.1155/2018/3931674. PMID: 30533242; PMCID: PMC6247711

[70] Kawaratani H, Matsumura M, Tsujimoto T, Morimoto T, Kitade M, Umemoto M, et al. A case of cardiac variceal rupture due to danaparoid sodium with portal venous thrombosis. Japanese Journal of Gastroenterology. 2008;**105**(12):1758-1765

[71] Kikuchi M, Nishizaki Y, Tsuruya K, Hamada I, Higashi T, Sakuma K, et al. Acute portal vein thrombosis due to chronic relapsing pancreatitis: A fistula between a pancreatic pseudocyst and the pancreatic vein. Clinical Journal of Gastroenterology. 2014;7:52-57

[72] Lefevre A, Soyer P, Vahedi K, Geurrache Y, Bellucci S, Gault V, et al. Multiple abdominal venous thrombosis in ulcerative colitis: Role of MDCT for detection. Clinical Imaging. 2011;**35**:68-72

[73] Matsuhashi N, Kunieda K, Yamada A, Sasaki Y, Tanaka C, Nishina T, et al. A patient with portal/superior mesenteric venous thrombosis in whom massive intestinal resection could be avoided by danaparoid sodium administration. J Jpn Soc Abdominal Emergency Med. 2010;**30**(1):65-68

[74] Nagato M, Goto K, Harayama N, Nihai S, Mouri F, Aibara K, et al. A case of portal vein thrombosis followed by sepsis successfully treated with danaparoid sodium and endotoxin absorption therapy. J Jpn Assoc Acute Med. 2009;**20**:126-132

[75] Nakajima Y, Takahashi A, Kanno Y, Gunji N, Imaizumi M, Hayashi M, et al. Paralytic ileus due to superior mesenteric thrombosis after transarterial injection for hepatocellular carcinoma. Internal Medicine. 2016;**55**(1):37-42

[76] Nawata Y, Hamada K, Tajima H, Nishino N, Nakazawa T, Tobayashi K, et al. Successful use of danaparoid in the treatment of portal vein thrombosis that developed in a warfarin administered hepatitis C virus-related cirrhosis patient. Japanese Journal of Gastroenterology. 2012;**109**(8):1394-1400

[77] Nomura H, Katsuramaki T, Tooru M, Hidefumi M, Kikuchi H, Koichi H. A case of portal vein thrombosis successfully treated with danaparoid sodium after splenectomy for massive splenomegaly. Journal of Jaffna Science Association. 2003;**64**(3):705-709

[78] Oguri H, Tanaka S, Kakuma K. A case of liver cirrhosis C recovered from portal vein thrombosis developed during chemotherapy of pancreatic cancer with antithrombin-III and danaparoid sodium. Kanzo. 2009;**50**:377-382

[79] Ohe M, Mutsuki K, Goya T, Yamashita S, Satoh T, Kojima M, et al. Portal vein thrombosis repeatedly observed in a cirrhotic patient with antiphospholipid antibody syndrome. Fukuoka Acta Medica. 2016;**107**(10):185-190

[80] Oku T, Kubo Y, Sakai T, Yamakawa A, Sugata H. A case of portal vein thrombosis complicating acute cholangitis treated successfully with danaparoid sodium. Journal of Japanese Society of Gastroenterology. 2010;**107**(11):1814-1820

[81] Roullet S, Biais M, Stecken L, Laurent C, Neau-Cransac M, SztarkF.rombocytopeniaandBudd-Chiari syndrome after liver transplantation: Heparin-induced thrombocytopenia. British Journal of Anaesthesia. 2011;**107**(3):475-477

[82] Shudo R, Yazaki Y, Sugawara K, Honda M. Treatment by danaparoid sodium for portal venous thrombosis. Nihon Shokakibyo Gakkai Zasshi. 2007;**104**(2):205-212

[83] Shudo R, Yazaki Y, Honda M, Sugawara M. A case in which danaparoid sodium was effective for portal vein thrombosis developed after endoscopic injection of sclerotherapy for esophageal varices. Clinical Journal of Gastroenterology. 2008;**1**(3):110-115

[84] Shigefuku R, Suzuki M, Kobayashi M, Michikawa Y, Hiraishi T, Ikeda H, et al. Three cases of liver abscess associated with the Streptococcus anginosus group. Japanese Journal of Gastroenterology. 2013;**110**(8):1468-1480

[85] Sugimoto A, Fukuoka T, Nagahara H, Shibutani M, Iseki Y, Ohira M. Danaparoid sodium effectively treats portal vein thrombosis after laparoscopic inter-sphincteric resection for rectal cancer: A case report. Nihon Rinsho Geka Gakkai Zasshi (Journal of Japan Surgical Association). 2020;**80**(8):1508-1512

[86] Takada H, Kurosaki M, Nakanishi H, Takahashi Y, Itakura K, Tsuchiya K, et al. Real-life experience of lusutrombopag for cirrhotic patients with low platelet counts being prepared for invasive procedures. PLoS One. Feb 15, 2019;**14**(2):e0211122. DOI: 10.1371/journal.pone.0211122. PMID: 30768601; PMCID: PMC6377090

[87] Tatsumi R, Ozeki I, Yamaguchi M, Kimura M, Arakawa T, Nakajima T, et al. A case of amebic liver abscess complicated by hepatic vein thrombus and pulmonary embolism. Acta Hepatologica Japonica. 2017;**58**(10):574-581

[88] Uchiyama T, Takahashi H, Hosono K, Endo H, Akiyama T, Yoneda K, et al. Portal vein thrombosis treated using danaparoid sodium and antithrombin III. Hepato-Gastroenterology. 2010;**57**:52-53

[89] Uehara H, Kawanaka H, Nakanoko T, Sugiyama M, Ota M, Mano Y, et al. Successful hybrid surgery for ileal conduit stomal varices following oxaliplatin-based chemotherapy in a patient with advanced colorectal cancer. Surgical Case Reports. 2020;**6**:236. DOI: 10.1186/s40792-020-01021-6

[90] Yokota K, Ishizu H, Kondo Y, Okada K, Masuko H, Yokota R. A case of portal vein thrombosis successfully treated with danaparoid sodium after splenectomy. Japan Surgical Society. 2005;**66**(4):899-903

[91] Bsilat M, Leonard D, van Nieuwenhove S, Lambert C. Portal trunk occlusion leading to small bowel resection in a context of pyelophlebitis complicated by heparin-induced thrombocytopenia. Louvain Medical (Hematologie). 2017;**136**(7):440-449

[92] Ito M, Saito S, Fujii M, Ishiyama S, Fujiwara A, Nasu J, Yoshioka M, Shiode J, Yamamoto K. Superior mesenteric thrombosis followed by gastric varices. Poster at 23rd UEG week (Barcelona). 2015

[93] Sakuma Y, Yazumi S, Fukunaga T, Yamamoto A, Hamuro M, Nakamura K. Melena from jejunal mucosal varices caused by esophageal variceal sclerotherapy-induced arteriovenous fistula. Gastrointestinal Endoscopy. 2011;**74**(2):404-405

[94] Sehgal M, Haskal ZJ. Use of transjugular intrahepatic portosystemic shunts during lytic therapy of extensive portal splenic and mesenteric venous thrombosis: Long term follow-up. Journal of Vascular and Interventional Radiology. 2000;**11**:61-65

[95] Cui SB, Shu RH, Yan SP, Wu H, Chen Y, Wang L, et al. Efficacy and safety of anticoagulation therapy with different doses of enoxaparin for portal vein thrombosis in cirrhosis patients with hepatitis B. European Journal of Gastroenterology & Hepatology. 2015;**27**:914-919

[96] Senzolo M, Garcia-Tsao G, Garcia-Pagan JC. Current knowledge and management of portal vein thrombosis in cirrhosis. Journal of Hepatology. 2021;**75**:442-453

[97] Francoz C, Valla D, Durand F. Portal vein thrombosis, cirrhosis, and liver transplantation. Journal of Hepatology. 2012;**57**:203-212

[98] Kwon J, Ko Y, Yu S-j, Yoon JH. Low-molecular-weight heparin treatment for portal vein thrombosis in liver cirrhosis: Efficacy and the risk of hemorrhagic complications. Thrombosis Research. 2018;**163**:71-76

[99] Pellicelli AM, D'Ambrioso C, Barbaro G, Villani R, Guarascio P, Fondacaro L, et al. Clinical and genetic factors associated to development of portal vein thrombosis in cirrhotic patients without hepatocellular carcinoma. Journal of Hepatology. 2011;**54**:S77 Abstract 180

[100] Amitrano L, Guardascione MA, Brancaccio V, et al. Risk factors and clinical presentation of portal vein thrombosis in patients with liver cirrhosis. Journal of Hepatology. 2004;**40**(5):736-741

[101] Bento L, Huerta A, Pascual C, et al. Antithrombotic therapy in non-neoplastic chronic portal venous thrombosis in cirrhosis: Recanalization and liver function evaluation. ASH Annual Meeting Abstracts. 2011;**118**:3358

[102] Chen H et al. Efficacy and safety of anticoagulation in more advanced portal vein thrombosis in patients with liver cirrhosis. European Journal of Gastroenterology & Hepatology. 2016;**28**(1):82-89

[103] Wang H, Kopac D, Brisebois R, Sample C, Shapiro AM. Randomized controlled trial to investigate the impact of anticoagulation on the incidence of splenic or portal vein thrombosis after laparoscopic splenectomy. Canadian Journal of Surgery. 2011;**54**:227-231

[104] Werner KT, Sando S, Carey EJ, et al. Portal vein thrombosis in patients with end stage liver disease awaiting liver transplantation: Outcome of anticoagulation. Digestive Diseases and Sciences. 2013;**58**:1776-1780

[105] Chung JW, Kim GF, Lee JH, Ok KS, Jang ES, Jeong S-H, et al. Safety, efficacy, and response predictors of anticoagulation for the treatment of nonmalignant portal-vein thrombosis in patients with cirrhosis: A propensity score matching analysis. Clinical and Molecular Hepatology. 2014;**20**(4):384-391. DOI: 10.3350/cmh.2014.20.4.384

[106] Cao G et al. Treatment of postoperative main portal vein and superior mesenteric vein thrombosis with balloon angioplasty and/or

stent placement. Acta Radiologica. 2013;**54**(5):526-532

[107] Copaci I, Ismail G, Micu L, et al. Anticoagulant therapy with sulodexidum for portal vein thrombosis in patients with liver cirrhosis. Hepatology. 2013;**58**:867A-868A

[108] Okamura H, Nishimoto M, Nakane T, Koh H, Nakashima Y, Takeoka Y, et al. Prophylactic use of a combination of an anticoagulant and ursodeoxycholic acid for sinusoidal obstruction syndrome after allogeneic myeloablative hematopoietic stem cell transplantation. Blood. 2016;**128**:5755

[109] Machida S, Onizuka M, Toyosaki M, Aoyama Y, Kawai H, Amaki J, et al. Danaparoid reduces the incidence of hematopoietic stem cell transplantation-associated thrombotic microangiopathy. Bone Marrow Transplantation. 2017;**52**(2):307-309

[110] Kato K, Sakaguchi H, Muramatsu H, Sekiya Y, Kawashima N, Narita A, et al. Danaparoid reduces transplant-related mortality in stem cell transplantation for children. Pediatric Transplantation. 2018;**22**(2). DOI: 10.1111/petr.13099. [Epub Dec 13, 2017]. PMID: 29239087

[111] Kato K, Maemura R, Wakamatsu M, Yamamori A, Hamada M, Kataoka S, et al. Allogeneic stem cell transplantation with reduced intensity conditioning for patients with adrenoleukodystrophy. Molecular Genetics and Metabolism Reports. 2019;**18**:1-6. DOI: 10.1016/j.ymgmr.2018.11.001

[112] Sakaguchi H, Maemura R, Yoshida N. Prophylaxis and treatment strategy for haematopoietic cell transplantation in children. Biology of Blood and Marrow Transplantation. 2019;**25**:S154 Abstract 211

[113] Yoshimura S, Kyotani C, Osumi T, Shioda Y, Terashima K, Kato M, et al. Pre-emptive treatment with recombinant thrombomodulin for children who developed veno-occlusive disease after hematopoietic stem cell transplantation: A single Centre experience. Pediatric Blood & Cancer. 2018;**65**(Suppl. 2):S18-S19

[114] Yoshida N, Sakaguchi H, Matsumoto K, Kato K. Successful treatment with low dose gemtuzumab ozogamicin-combined chemotherapy followed by unrelated stem-cell transplantation for children with refractory acute myeloid leukaemia. British Journal of Haematology. 2012;**158**(5):666-668

[115] Kojima Y, Maeoka E, Nisaka Y, Fukushima Y, Hashimoto T, Satou A, et al. A case of late onset veno-occlusive disease after hematopoietic stem cell transplantation in which ultrasonography was useful for the diagnosis and follow-up. Jpn J Med Ultrasonics (Choonpa Igaku). 2020;**166**. DOI: 10.3179/jjmu.JJMU.A.166

[116] Bidlingmaier C, Magnani HN, Girisch M, Kurnik K. Safety and efficacy of danaparoid (Orgaran®) use in children. Acta Haematologica. 2006;**115**(3-4):237-247

[117] Tay J, Tinmouth A, Fergusson D, Huebsch L, Allan DS. Systematic review of controlled clinical trials on the use of ursodeoxycholic acid for the prevention of hepatic veno-occlusive disease in hematopoietic stem cell transplantation. Biology of Blood and Marrow Transplantation. 2007;**13**:206-217

[118] Ohashi K, Tanabe J, Watanabe R, Tanaka T, Sakamaki H, Maruta A, et al. The Japanese multicenter open randomized trial of ursodeoxycholic acid prophylaxis for hepatic veno-occlusive

disease after stem cell transplantation. American Journal of Hematology. 2000;**64**:32-38

[119] Ruutu T, Eriksson B, Remes K, Juvonen E, Volin L, Remberger M, et al. Ursodeoxycholic acid for the prevention of hepatic complications in allogeneic stem cell transplantation. Blood. 2002;**100**:1977-1983

[120] Park SH, Lee MH, Lee H, Kim HS, Kim K, Kim WS, et al. A randomized trial of heparin plus ursodiol vs. heparin alone to prevent hepatic veno-occlusive disease after hematopoietic stem cell transplantation. Bone Marrow Transplantation. 2002;**29**:137-143

[121] Corbacioglu S, Cesaro S, Faraci M, Valteau-Couanet D, Gruhn B, Rovelli A, et al. Defibrotide for prophylaxis of hepatic veno-occlusive disease in paediatric haemopoietic stem-cell transplantation: An open-label, phase 3, randomised controlled trial. Lancet. 2012;**379**:1301-1309

[122] Essell JH, Schroeder MT, Harman GS, Halvorson R, Lew V, Callander N, et al. Ursodiol prophylaxis against hepatic complications of allogeneic bone marrow transplantation. A randomized, double-blind, placebo-controlled trial. Annals of Internal Medicine. 1998;**128**:975-981

[123] Zhang L, Wang Y, Huang H. Defibrotide for the prevention of hepatic veno-occlusive disease after haematopoietic stem-cell transplantation: A systemic review. Clinical Transplantation. 2012;**26**:511-519

[124] Higham CS, Melton A, Kharbanda S, Dara J, Winestone LE, Huang JN, et al. A pilot trial of pre-transplant risk stratification and prophylactic defibrotide to prevent serious thrombotic microangiopathy in high-risk pediatric hematopoietic stem cell transplant patients. Blood. 2020;**136**(Suppl 1):9-10

[125] Rothschedl E, Nachtnebel A. Defibrotide for the treatment and prophylaxis of hepatic veno-occlusive disease. Decision support document No. 84; Vienna: Ludwig Boltzmann for Health Technology Assessment2015

[126] Richardson PG, Carreras E, Iacobelli M, Nejadnik B. The use of defibrotide in blood and marrow transplantation. Blood Advances. 2018;**2**(12):1195-1509. DOI: 10.1182/bloodadvances.2017008375

[127] Chalandon YC, Simonetta F, Dantin C, Koutsi A, Mamez A-C, Beauverd Y, et al. Efficient prophylaxis with defibrotide for sinusoidal obstruction syndrome (SOS) after allogeneic hematopoietic stem cell transplantation (HSCT). Blood. 2016;**128**(22):2204-2207. DOI: 10.1182/blood.V128.22.2204.2204

[128] Richardson PG, Smith AR, Triplett BM, Kernan NA, Grupp SA, Antin JH, et al. Earlier defibrotide initiation post diagnosis of veno-occlusive disease/sinusoidal obstruction syndrome improves day + 100 survival following haemopoietic stem cell transplantation. British Journal of Haematology. 2017;**178**:112-118. DOI: 10.1111/bjh.14727

[129] Kayikci O, Akpinar S, Tekgunduz E. Effectiveness of defibrotide in the prevention of hepatic veno-occlusive disease among adult patients receiving allogeneic hematopoietic cell transplantation: A retrospective single center experience. Transfus Apher Sci. Feb 2022;**61**(1):103369. DOI: 10.1016/j.transci.2022.103369. [Epub Jan 24, 2022]. PMID: 35120824

[130] Corbacioglu S, Aggarwal S, Topaloglu O, Tappe W. A systematic study of defibrotide prophylaxis of veno-occlusive disease/sinusoidal obstruction syndrome. Biol. Bone Marrow Transplantation. 2020;**26**:S133 Abstract 187

[131] Picod A, Bonnin A, Battiplagia G, Giannotti F, Ruggeri A, Brissot E, et al. Defibrotide for sinusoidal obstruction syndrome/neo occlusive disease prophylaxis in high risk patients: A single-center experience study. Biology of Blood and Marrow Transplantation. 2018;**24**:1471-1475. DOI: 10.1016/j.bbmt.201802.015

[132] Kojima S, Watanabe N, Koizumi J, Kokubu S, Murashima N, Matsutani S, et al. Current status of portal vein thrombosis in Japan: Results of a questionnaire survey by the Japanese Society for Portal Vein Thrombosis. Hepatology Research. 2018;**48**(4): 244-254. DOI: 10.1111/hepr.12983

[133] Magnani HN, Gallus A. Heparin induced thrombocytopenia: A report of 1478 clinical outcomes of patients treated with danaparoid (Orgaran®) from 1982 to mid-2004. Thrombosis and Haemostasis. 2006;**95**(6):967-968

[134] Tagami T, Matsui H, Horiguchi H, Fushimi K, Yasunaga H. Recombinant human thrombomodulin and mortality in severe pneumonia patients with sepsis associated disseminated intravascular coagulation: An observational study. Journal of Thrombosis and Haemostasis. 2015;**13**:31-40

[135] Yoshihara H, Sugiura-Ogasawara M, Kitaori T, Katano K, Ozaki Y. Danaparoid is effective and safe for patients with obstetric antiphospholipid syndrome. Modern Rheumatology. 2020;**30**(2):332-337. DOI: 10.1080/14397595.2019.1602241

[136] Katano K, Sugiura M. Danaparoid versus heparin therapy in recurrent pregnancy loss patients with antiphospholipid syndrome. Fertility Sterility. 2011;**96**(3 Suppl. 1):S283 Abstract P-594

[137] de Guibert S, Peffault de Latour R, Varoqueaux N, Labussiere H, Rio B, Jaulmes D, et al. Paroxysmal nocturnal haemoglobinuria and pregnancy before the eculizumab era: The French experience. Haematologica. 2011;**96**(9):1276-1283

[138] Bhavnani K. Jazz pharmaceuticals stops enrolment in Phase 3 study evaluating defibrotide for the prevention of veno-occlusive disease. News release. April 2020. https://investor.jazzpharma.com/news-release//news-release-details/j

[139] Pichler H, Horner K, Engstler G, Poetschger U, Glogova E, Karlhuber S, et al. Cost effectiveness of defibrotide in the prophylaxis of veno-occlusive disease after paediatric allogeneic stem cell transplantation. Biology of Blood and Marrow Transplantation. 2017;**23**(7):1128-1133. DOI: 10.1016/j.bbmt.2017.03

[140] Boberg KM, Wisloff T, Kjollesdal KS, Stovring H, Kistiansen IS. Cost and health consequences of treatment of primary biliary cirrhosis with ursodeoxycholic acid. Alimentary Pharmacology & Therapeutics. 2013;**38**:794-803

Chapter 5

COVID-19 and Thrombosis: Pathophysiological Mechanisms and Therapeutic Update

Isabel Izuzquiza-Avanzini, Raquel Gutiérrez-López, Manuel Lorenzo López-Reboiro, Clara Martínez-Vivero and José López-Castro

Abstract

Severe acute respiratory syndrome coronavirus 2 (SARS-CoV-2) is a pro-inflammatory and prothrombogenic virus with a high mutagenic profile, which produces active infection of variable duration in various organs and systems, and it has been observed that patients who have already suffered from the disease, especially in its more severe forms such as bilateral pneumonia or respiratory distress, present symptoms and signs of chronic multi-organ involvement. However, little is known about the molecular mechanisms that generate endothelial damage (chronic reactive endotheliitis) and subsequent thrombosis in SARS-CoV-2 infection are still not sufficiently elucidated, and in this chapter, we explore these mechanisms and therapeutic options to reduce prothrombosis and multiple vascular involvement that cause morbidity and mortality in this disease. In particular, we will evaluate heparin doses according to the stage of infection and its correlation with improved survival.

Keywords: thrombosis, COVID-19, pathophysiology, heparin, mortality

1. Introduction

SARS-CoV-2 causing coronavirus disease (COVID-19) is a proinflammatory and prothrombogenic virus with a high mutation rate, producing active infection of variable duration in various organs and systems [1, 2]. The disease is highly heterogeneous in its manifestations and, although in most cases resolve asymptomatically or mildly, it can lead to severe symptoms and even death [3, 4]. In hospitalised patients with COVID-19, due to the procoagulant state and the increased risk of thromboembolic events, the use of anticoagulation for prophylactic purposes is recommended [5], and heparin is of great benefit in the treatment and prevention of venous and arterial micro- and macro-thrombosis [6]. Given reports of excess thrombotic risk, dose-escalating anticoagulation strategies have been incorporated into some COVID-19 clinical guidelines [7].

However, the effectiveness and safety of therapeutic/intermediate/prophylactic anticoagulation doses in COVID-19 are uncertain and remain under study [8].

2. Pathophysiology of the disease

2.1 Angiotensin-converting enzyme 2 receptor interaction

Angiotensin-converting enzyme 2 (ACE2) has been identified as a functional receptor for coronaviruses [6]. The ACE2 receptor is present throughout multiple cellular organs such as the heart, kidney, lungs, as well as in the central and peripheral nervous system [9]. As with other respiratory viruses, respiratory tract symptoms are the most common. The gradient of receptor expression has been directly correlated with the ability of SARS-CoV-2 to infect cells throughout the respiratory tract. The highest concentration of ACE2 receptors is found in the hair cells of the nasal mucosa and is 80% lower in trachea, bronchi and lung tissue [10]. SARS-CoV-2 binds to the transmembrane ACE2 protein to enter type II pneumocytes; due to this tropism, SARS-CoV-2 can interact with a large area of the pulmonary microvasculature. In addition, it can infect pericytes and perivascular cells on the surface of microvessels. ACE2 receptor expression on endothelial cells increases their vulnerability to SARS-CoV-2 binding, causing infection and subsequent vascular injury, dysfunction and endotheliitis [6]. Likewise, interaction with ACE2 receptors in the peripheral nervous system may contribute to the development of myopathies and neuropathies [9].

2.2 COVID-19-associated coagulopathy (CAC)

Most critically ill patients with COVID-19 present with isolated respiratory failure, usually acute respiratory distress syndrome (ARDS). In COVID-19 deaths, the predominant lung damage is diffuse alveolar damage, which includes hyaline membrane formation, capillary congestion, inflammation and pneumocyte necrosis [4, 11]. In addition, fibrin-platelet thrombi in small arterial vessels are also identified in many of these cases [4]. However, about 20–30% of these patients have multi-organ involvement. Among the extra respiratory complications present in COVID-19 are vascular alterations, among which coagulopathies are of great relevance [2]. In general, COVID-19-associated coagulopathy (CAC) is characterised by moderate thrombocytopenia, mildly increased prothrombin time (PT), elevated D-dimer and fibrinogen levels [4].

2.2.1 Chronic reactive endotheliitis and von Willebrand factor

There are different prothrombotic mechanisms in SARS-CoV-2 infection. It has been established that the virus induces oxidative stress at the endothelial level, causing the release of von Willebrand factor (vWF) multimers causing hypercoagulability, despite the thrombopenia caused by the virus, leading to a state of prothrombosis through increased thrombin and D-dimer levels [4, 12–14]. Thus, vWF may be implicated in CAC, due to its direct relationship with homeostasis, inflammation and endothelial cell activation and damage [4]. vWF is a large multimeric glycoprotein whose gene is located on the short arm of chromosome 12 at position 13.3 and has a length of 180 kb and 52 exons [15]. The VWF gene belongs to the endogenous ligand gene family and genetic differences between individuals are associated with vWF levels. This includes polymorphisms in the 5′ homeostatic factor regulatory region, which contributes to the level of vWF present in plasma and, consequently, to the risk of thrombotic events [15]. This protein is present in blood plasma, platelet-α-granules, subendothelial connective tissue and endothelium [4, 15]. vWF is synthesised and stored primarily in endothelial cells, megakaryocytes and platelet precursors in the bone marrow [15]. Upon synthesis in endothelial cells, the sequence of the vWF propeptide acts by aligning the 2 units of the molecule to ensure optimal multimerisation. Post-translational modifications involve the removal of the propeptide, glycosylation and the addition of blood group determinants, and then, a multitude of ultra-long vWF (UL-vWF) molecules are synthesised. When endothelial cells are activated, UL-vWF molecules are released and can remain free in plasma or bound to the endothelial surface. UL-vWF molecules exhibit greater prothrombotic activity than smaller vWF multiples. Simultaneously to the release of UL-vWF molecules, ADAMTS-13 (thrombospondin type 1 metalloprotease, member 13) cleaves these molecules into smaller multimers, to stop unwanted thrombus formation [4, 15]. This protein has a functional duality, as it is involved in both homeostasis and thrombosis [4, 15].

vWF plays a major role in primary haemostasis. When damage to the vascular wall occurs, the subendothelium to which vWF is bound is exposed. This protein interacts with platelets and promotes the recruitment of circulating platelets to the site of damage. Platelet-vWF binding is an adhesive interaction capable of binding platelets to the endothelial surface. Although the binding between platelets and vWF is unstable, it promotes a stronger and prolonged adhesion to the endothelium, which is mediated primarily by vWF [4, 15]. As for the process of secondary haemostasis, vWF also plays an important role and that process involves coagulation factors and the coagulation cascade to produce fibrin networks in areas of vascular damage. vWF promotes the process of secondary haemostasis by two mechanisms: Firstly, vWF acts as a transporter of coagulation factor VIII, stabilising it and extending its half-life in plasma. Secondly, it releases and concentrates factor VIII at the site of endothelial damage. Factor VIII is a coagulation factor that, when activated, complements other factors to generate fibrin [4].

During the inflammatory process, different mediators are released as inflammatory molecules activate endothelial cells to release their contents, such as vWF. UL-vWF molecules that remain attached to the cell surface will bind to platelets and serve as a surface to interact with leukocytes. Inflammation also promotes association between vWF molecules, leading to an increase in platelet adhesiveness and a decrease in ADAMTS-13 cleavage. In addition, high-density lipoprotein (HDL) levels decrease during the inflammatory process. HDL plays a key role in preventing the association of vWF molecules with inflammation, as well as decreasing the risk of thrombus under normal circumstances. Increased release of vWF can induce a prothrombotic state [4], which is a pathological state of the haemostatic process. Thrombi are composed of numerous elements including endothelial cells, plasma, proteins and alterations in haemodynamic stress [15]. There is evidence of an association between increased levels of vWF and increased risk of thrombosis [4, 16]; therefore during the inflammatory process, there is an increased risk of thrombosis due to the imbalance in which vWF level and activity are elevated due to over-activation of endothelial cells.

The increase in vWF levels in COVID-19 could be due to the release of this molecule from pulmonary endothelial cells as a result of the pathophysiological process of COVID-19 itself. Infection of endothelial cells by SARS-CoV-2 or their activation in response to inflammatory mediators results in the release of prothrombotic factors, such as vWF. vWF either binds to endothelial cells or circulates in plasma to promote platelet aggregation and thrombus formation (**Figure 1**) [4].

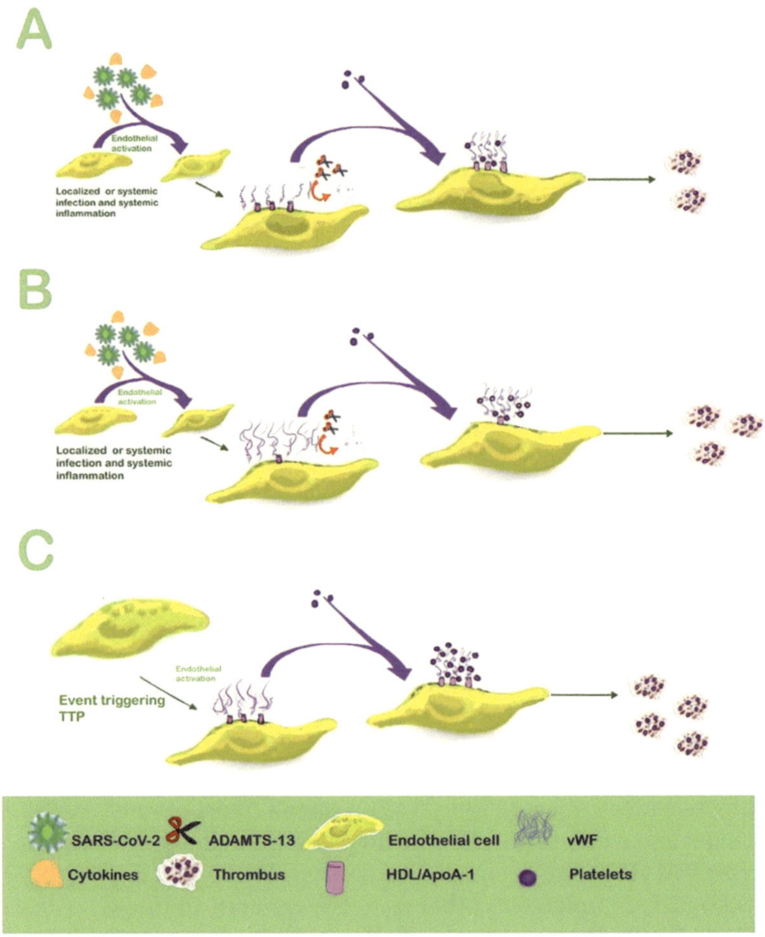

Figure 1.
Adapted from Mei et al., J. Appl. Lab. Med. 2021: Mechanism and characteristics of CAC in mild and severe cases. (A) CAC in mild cases. Localised infection and minimal systemic inflammation increase endothelial cell activation. Infection and inflammation remain well regulated. HDL and ADAMTS-13 mechanisms remain largely unchanged, with only a slight increase in thrombotic events. (B) CAC in severe cases. Infection and inflammation are deregulated, leading to an extremely high level of activated endothelial cells. In addition, HDL and ADAMTS-13 levels are decreased, leading to a much greater increase in thrombotic events. (C) Thrombotic thrombocytopenic Purpura (TTP). In TTP, ADAMTS-13 activity levels are significantly lower than in CAC. TTP leads to the elevated levels of UL-vWF. Consequently, platelet-binding levels increase and, consequently, the risk of thrombosis increases. Addendum: In the NIH COVID-19 treatment guidelines panel's statement on anticoagulation in hospitalized patients with COVID-19, last updated the 5th of January 2022, the panel recommends using therapeutic-dose heparin for patients who have a D-dimer above the upper limit of normal, require low-flow oxygen, and have no increased bleeding risk. They recommend continue therapeutic-dose heparin treatment for 14 days or until hospital discharge, whichever comes first [17].

2.2.2 Other agents: immunocomplexes, lupus anticoagulants, β-2 glycoprotein 1 (B2GPI) and cytokines

The proinflammatory and prothrombotic state at the endothelial level in the microvasculature may remain in some patients due to immunocomplex formation, causing chronic reactive endotheliitis with multiple vascular involvement, especially in the lungs and central nervous system (**Figure 2**) [13].

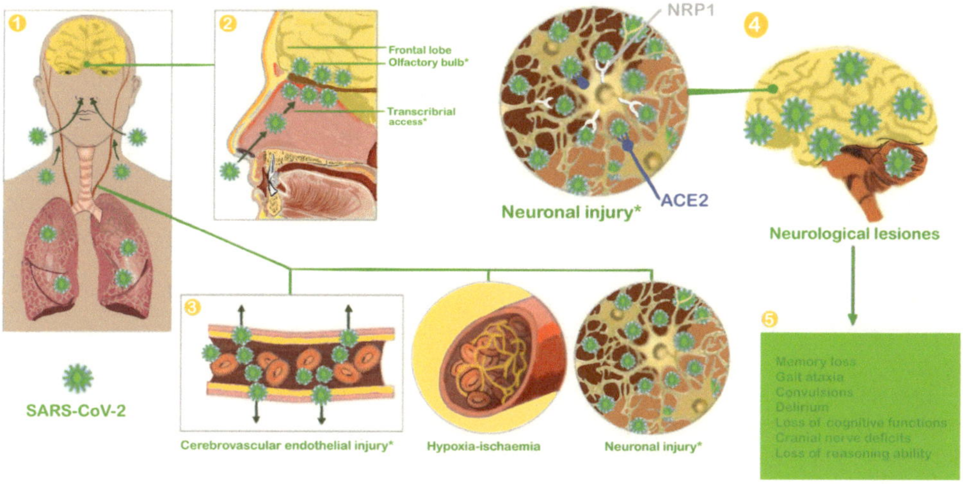

Figure 2.
Neurological lesions mediated by chronic reactive endotheliitis and multiple vascular involvement.

On the one hand, the presence of direct neurological damage by SARS-CoV-2 through the advancement into the CNS from the periphery *via* retrograde and trans-synaptic neuronal transport, especially *via* vagus nerve afferent pathways, has been demonstrated. Supported by the increasing findings that SARS CoV-2 infects cells in the gastrointestinal tract, the neuroinvasive potential could even encompass the enteric nervous system [18].

On the other hand, the pivotal role of lupus anticoagulants (LA) in the thrombogenesis of SARS-CoV-2 has also been observed [19, 20] and an increased prothrombin time has been reported in COVID-19 patients. This may be indicative of a coagulation factor deficiency or the presence of an inhibitor, either specific such as the factor VIII antibody or non-specific like LA [20]. The β-2 glycoprotein 1 (B2GPI), involved in thrombogenesis, promotes LA activity, thereby stimulating platelet adhesion, tissue factor release and subsequent activation of the coagulation cascade, leading to an often irreversible prothrombotic state in advanced stages [19]. Ultimately, cytokine storm and immune abnormalities also contribute to the inflammatory process. These immune abnormalities have been associated with the severity of COVID-19 and are considered a cause of mortality in this disease [3, 11, 19]. A correlation between severe COVID-19 and abnormalities in circulating immune cells has been described [3]. In severe cases, COVID-19 can trigger an excessive immune response known as a cytokine storm, which is potentially fatal. It is characterised by over-activation of immune cells and excessive production of pro-inflammatory cytokines and chemical mediators [11]. Cytokine storm also amplifies platelet production, leading to an increased formation of disseminated microthrombi in various vascular territories, and is directly involved in the pathogenesis of thrombosis in this disease [19].

2.2.3 Immune response and T lymphocytes

In viral infections, "innocent bystander" activation of CD8+ T cells occurs, which consists of activation of CD8+ memory cells independent of T-cell receptor (TCR) stimulation. Active lymphocytes can migrate to the site of infection and kill infected cells. This form of early response, which begins before symptoms develop, may be associated with disease resolution and avoid progression to severe disease. However, persistent bystander activation of CD8+ T cells has been associated with inflammatory pathology in both chronic infections and autoimmune processes. Therefore, it is possible that persistent T cell activation in severe COVID-19 may influence the development of lung pathology and autoimmune manifestations observed in this disease [3]. On the other hand, patients with more severe clinical manifestations have higher-circulating TNF-α and IL-6, and higher gene expression of proinflammatory pathways [3, 11].

3. Therapeutic proposals: antithrombotic treatment

The recognition of thrombosis as a key contributor to clinical deterioration and death has led to a worldwide interest in the study of optimal antithrombotic treatment doses for patients. Clinical trials have shown that the efficacy and safety of these treatments vary according to the time course of the disease [21]. For this reason, treatment should be started early in the Emergency Department in all hospitalised patients and assessed according to thrombotic and haemorrhagic risk factors [22]. Haematological and coagulation parameters (e.g. D-dimer, prothrombin time, platelet count, fibrinogen) are commonly measured. Evidence shows that elevated D-dimer values correlate positively with disease severity and prognosis [23]. However, at present, there is insufficient evidence to recommend for or against the use of these data to guide management decisions [7, 24]. Dosing recommendations are dynamic and have changed throughout the pandemic. The results of recent scientific publications have generated controversy about the best strategy for antithrombotic prophylaxis and treatment, which is reflected in the variability of consensus recommendations published by different scientific organisations and societies [25]. In terms of treatment, we differentiate between non-hospitalised and hospitalised patients.

3.1 Non-hospitalised patients

For non-hospitalised patients with COVID-19, antithrombotic therapy or antiplatelet therapy for the prevention of venous thromboembolism (VTE) or arterial thrombosis should not be initiated unless the patient has other indications for therapy (prior PTE or DVT, recent surgery, trauma or immobilisation) or is participating in a clinical trial. Patients with COVID-19 receiving warfarin/acenocoumarol who are isolated and therefore unable to proceed with standardised monitoring of anticoagulation levels may be candidates for switching to direct oral anticoagulation therapy [26].

3.2 Patients hospitalised for COVID-19

All patients hospitalised with COVID-19 should receive prophylactic dose antithrombotic therapy with low-molecular-weight heparin unless contraindicated (e.g. active bleeding or severe thrombocytopenia) [7, 26]. Low-molecular-weight (LMW) heparin is preferred, but unfractionated heparin may be used if LMW heparin is not available or if renal function is severely impaired (creatinine clearance <30 ml/min). Individuals with a history of heparin-induced thrombocytopenia (HIT) or active HIT should not receive low-molecular-weight heparin or unfractionated heparin; instead, Fondaparinux is advised. Aspirin is not indicated outside the usual standard indications [7, 26]. Patients chronically receiving anticoagulant or antiplatelet therapies for underlying conditions should continue these medications unless they have a bleeding or contraindication to them. In patients on chronic anticoagulant therapy, heparin is preferable to oral anticoagulants because of its shorter half-life, the possibility of intravenous or subcutaneous administration, and the reduced presence of drug interactions [26]. In addition, it has antithrombotic, anti-inflammatory and possibly antiviral properties [27].

In the case of suspected venous thromboembolic disease in patients with COVID-19, the recommendations proposed by the scientific societies for any patient with suspected and confirmed thrombotic disease should be followed [7, 26].
For most hospitalised patients with COVID-19, prophylactic dosing is supported. However, following the publication of several large and well-conducted randomised trials, the relative benefits of prophylactic, intermediate or therapeutic dosing continue to generate debate [28]. This is partly due to the increased risk of bleeding attributed to intermediate and therapeutic regimens [29].

Within inpatients, we differentiate those with moderate/non-critical illness from those with critical illness.

3.2.1 Moderately ill or non-critically ill patients

Patients with moderate/non-critical illness are those with clinical features that would normally result in admission to an inpatient ward without the need for advanced clinical support in intensive care unit (ICU). Examples include patients with mild to moderate dyspnoea or hypoxia [5, 21]. In recent months, several randomised clinical trials (ACTIV-4, REMAP-CAP and ATTACC, RAPID and HEP COVID) have shown that in non-critically ill hospitalised patients with COVID-19, heparin at therapeutic doses may be beneficial, with a high probability of reducing the need for organ support and progression to intubation and death [26, 30, 31]. Other trials, however (ACTION, BEMICOP), found no benefit in therapeutic versus prophylactic dosing [32, 33]. The multi-platform randomised clinical trial (ACTIV-4, REMAP-CAP and ATTACC) showed that in non-critically ill hospitalised patients with COVID-19, an initial strategy of therapeutic anticoagulation with heparin increased the likelihood of survival to hospital discharge with a reduced need for ICU-level organ support at 21 days compared with usual care thromboprophylaxis. Therapeutic dose anticoagulation was beneficial regardless of the patient's baseline D-dimer level. Therapeutic anticoagulation was administered according to local protocols for the treatment of acute venous thromboembolism for up to 14 days or until recovery. The need for organ support was defined as the need for high-flow nasal oxygen, invasive or non-invasive mechanical ventilation, vasopressor therapy or extracorporeal membrane oxygenation (ECMO) [30]. A subsequent randomised clinical trial (RAPID) demonstrated that the use of therapeutic heparin in moderately ill patients with COVID-19 and increased D-dimer levels (above the upper limit set by the local laboratory) were not associated with a significant reduction in the primary composite outcome of death, non-invasive or invasive mechanical ventilation, or ICU admission. However, it decreased the probability of death at 28 days and showed a low risk of haemorrhage [31]. Finally, in the randomised HEP-COVID clinical trial, therapeutic-dose LMWH in hospitalised COVID-19 patients with D-dimer levels at least four times the upper limit of normal reduced the outcome of thromboembolism and death at 30 days compared with standard heparin thromboprophylaxis, without increasing the risk of major bleeding [34]. The effectiveness of anticoagulation appears to depend on the type of anticoagulant; for example, the Coronavirus Anticoagulation Trial (ACTION) used 15–20 mg rivaroxaban in 94% of patients assigned to therapeutic anticoagulation and found no benefit [32]. Finally, the randomised controlled clinical trial BEMICOP randomised adult patients with non-critical COVID and elevated D-dimer to receive heparin at therapeutic versus prophylactic doses for 10 days; however, the use of a short course of heparin at therapeutic doses did not improve the primary outcome (death, death in the intensive care unit), intensive care unit admission, need for mechanical ventilation support, the development of moderate/severe acute respiratory distress and venous or arterial thrombosis) over the subsequent 10 days compared with the use of heparin at a prophylactic dose [33].

In view of the discordance in different clinical trials, recent meta-analyses have attempted to clarify whether higher dosing (intermediate or therapeutic) could be of benefit over prophylactic dosing. Both groups of studies, the ones that included cohort studies and clinical trials [35], as well as those that included only randomised clinical trials [24, 28], have shown that higher anticoagulation dose (intermediate or therapeutic) is not associated with lower in-hospital mortality or incidence of thrombotic events, but increases the risk of bleeding events. There is currently insufficient evidence of survival benefit of therapeutic or intermediate dose anticoagulation compared with prophylactic dose anticoagulation in hospitalised patients with COVID-19.

The meta-analysis by Jorda et al. [24] included 10 randomised controlled open-label trials with a total of 5753 patients. The risk of death was similar between therapeutic dose versus prophylactic dose anticoagulation (RR 0.92, 95% CI 0.69–1.21, P = 0.54) and between intermediate dose versus prophylactic dose anticoagulation (RR 1.01, 95% CI 0.63–1.61, P = 0.98). In patients with markedly increased D-dimer levels, higher-dose anticoagulation was also not associated with a lower risk of death compared with prophylactic dose anticoagulation (RR 0.86, 95% CI 0.64–1.16, P = 0.34). In the meta-analysis by Ortega Paz L et al. [28] including seven randomised controlled trials with 5154 patients, prophylactic dose-escalated anticoagulation was not associated with a reduction in all-cause death [17.8% vs. 18.6%, hazard ratio (HR) 0.96, 95% confidence interval (CI) 0.78–1.18], but was associated with an increase in major haemorrhage.

In conclusion, the literature that has so far been published provides evidence for the use of prophylactic anticoagulation at standard doses over a dose-escalating regimen in routine care for patients hospitalised for COVID-19, irrespective of disease severity. There may be a subgroup of patients with moderate disease where heparin at therapeutic doses may be beneficial; however, further studies are needed to define this subgroup of patients.

3.2.2 Severely ill/critically ill patients

Patients with severe/critical COVID-19-related illness are those requiring respiratory or cardiovascular support (oxygen *via* high-flow nasal cannula, non-invasive or invasive mechanical ventilation, extracorporeal life support, vasopressors or inotropes) usually in an intensive care unit [5]. For thromboprophylaxis in critically ill hospitalised COVID-19 patients, prophylactic dosing is recommended rather than more intensive (intermediate or therapeutic) dosing. Randomised trials published to date have not consistently demonstrated better outcomes with more intensive dosing in critically ill patients, but have found an association with a higher likelihood of side effects (bleeding) and most institutions have adopted prophylactic dosing standards [7]. In the multi-platform ACTIV-4, REMAP-CAP and ATTACC study, a parallel analysis of the same trial mentioned above, in patients with COVID-19 critical illness, empirical anticoagulation at therapeutic doses was not beneficial in this group of patients [8]. Nor did heparin at anticoagulant doses show benefit in the group of critically ill patients in the HEP-COVID study [34]. The randomised clinical trial (INSPIRATION) in critically ill patients with COVID-19 showed no benefit of intermediate-dose heparin either [36]. Patients with COVID-19 who require ECMO or continuous renal replacement therapy or who have catheter or extracorporeal filter thrombosis should be treated according to standard institutional protocols for non-COVID-19 patients [26].

4. Conclusions

COVID-19 is associated with a hypercoagulable state with acute inflammatory changes. Fibrinogen and D-dimer are increased, with a typical mild prolongation of prothrombin time (PT) and modest thrombocytopenia. The pathogenesis of these abnormalities is not fully understood, and there may be many other related factors contributing to the acute inflammatory response to the disease. Routine thromboprophylactic medication is not recommended in outpatients. For thromboprophylaxis in hospitalised patients with COVID-19, prophylactic antithrombotic dosing with low-molecular-weight heparin is recommended in both moderately and critically ill patients. There may be a subgroup of patients with moderate disease where heparin at therapeutic doses could be beneficial in reducing the need for organ support and death; however, further studies are needed to precisely define this subgroup of patients due to heterogeneity of results.

In critically ill patients, randomised trials with intensive dosing have shown no benefit, but an increased risk of bleeding.

Acknowledgements

The authors wish to express their great gratitude to Mrs. Charo Ibáñez González, secretary of the Internal Medicine Department for all these years shared and for her great dedication to the continuous improvement of the Department.

Conflict of interest

The authors declare that they have no conflicts of interest.

Author details

Isabel Izuzquiza-Avanzini[1], Raquel Gutiérrez-López[2],
Manuel Lorenzo López-Reboiro[2], Clara Martínez-Vivero[2] and José López-Castro[2]*

1 Internal Medicine Dep. Hospital Universitario de Ourense, Ourense, Spain

2 Internal Medicine Dep. Hospital Público de Monforte, Lugo, Spain

*Address all correspondence to: jlcastro126@hotmail.com

References

[1] López CJ. Post-COVID-19 syndrome (PC19S): Chronic reactive endothelitis and disseminated vascular disease. Acta Médica Portuguesa. 2020;**33**(12):855

[2] Colling ME, Kanthi Y. COVID–19-associated coagulopathy: An exploration of mechanisms. Vascular Medicine. 2020;**25**(5):471-478

[3] Bergamaschi L, Mescia F, Turner L, Hanson AL, Kotagiri P, Dunmore BJ, et al. Longitudinal analysis reveals that delayed bystander CD8+ T cell activation and early immune pathology distinguish severe COVID-19 from mild disease. Immunity. 2021;**54**(6):1257-1275.e8. Available from: http://www.ncbi.nlm.nih.gov/pubmed/34051148

[4] Mei ZW, van Wijk XMR, Pham HP, Marin MJ. Role of von Willebrand factor in COVID-19 associated coagulopathy. The Journal of Applied Laboratory Medicine. 2021;**6**(5):1305-1315. Available from: http://www.ncbi.nlm.nih.gov/pubmed/33930144

[5] Cuker A, Tseng EK, Nieuwlaat R, Angchaisuksiri P, Blair C, Dane K, et al. American society of hematology 2021 guidelines on the use of anticoagulation for thromboprophylaxis in patients with COVID-19. Blood Advances. 2021;**5**(3):872-888

[6] Ortega-Paz L, Capodanno D, Montalescot G, Angiolillo DJ. Coronavirus disease 2019–associated thrombosis and coagulopathy: Review of the pathophysiological characteristics and implications for antithrombotic management. Journal of the American Heart Association. 2021;**10**(3):1-24

[7] National Institute for Health and Care Excellence. COVID-19 rapid guideline: Managing COVID-19. National Institute for Health and Care Excellence. 2021:1-78. Available from: https://www.nice.org.uk/guidance/ng191/resources/covid19-rapid-guideline-managing-covid19-pdf-51035553326

[8] REMAP-CAP Investigators, ACTIV-4a Investigators, ATTACC Investigators, Goligher EC, Bradbury CA, McVerry BJ, et al. Therapeutic anticoagulation with heparin in critically ill patients with Covid-19. The New England Journal of Medicine. 2021;**385**(9):777-789. Available from: http://www.ncbi.nlm.nih.gov/pubmed/34351722

[9] Fiani B, Covarrubias C, Desai A, Sekhon M, Jarrah R. A contemporary review of neurological sequelae of COVID-19. Frontiers in Neurology. 2020;**11**:1-9

[10] Hou YJ, Okuda K, Edwards CE, Martinez DR, Asakura T, Dinnon KH, et al. SARS-CoV-2 reverse genetics reveals a variable infection gradient in the respiratory tract. Cell. 2020;**182**(2):429-446.e14

[11] Hu B, Huang S, Yin L. The cytokine storm and COVID-19. Journal of Medical Virology. 2021;**93**(1):250-256. Available from: http://www.ncbi.nlm.nih.gov/pubmed/32592501

[12] Sieiro-Santos C, López-Castro J. Post-coronavirus disease syndrome and disseminated microthrombosis: The role of the von Willebrand factor and antiphospholipid antibodies. Clinics (Sao Paulo). 2021;**76**:e2784. Available from: https://www.ncbi.nlm.nih.gov/pmc/articles/PMC7955146/

[13] López CJ. Approach to post-COVID-19 syndrome (PC19S): How long to maintain corticotherapy and heparin after discharge

from intensive care? Revista Española de Geriatría y Gerontología. 2021;**56**(6):380. Available from: http://www.ncbi.nlm.nih.gov/pubmed/34154837

[14] Falcinelli E, Petito E, Becattini C, De Robertis E, Paliani U, Sebastiano M, et al. Role of endothelial dysfunction in the thrombotic complications of COVID-19 patients. The Journal of Infection. 2021;**82**(5):186-230. Available from: http://www.ncbi.nlm.nih.gov/pubmed/33275957

[15] Shahidi M. Thrombosis and von Willebrand factor. Advances in Experimental Medicine and Biology. 2017;**906**:285-306. Available from: http://www.ncbi.nlm.nih.gov/pubmed/27628010

[16] Jansson JH, Nilsson TK, Johnson O. von Willebrand factor in plasma: A novel risk factor for recurrent myocardial infarction and death. Heart. 1991;**66**(5):351-355. Available from: https://heart.bmj.com/lookup/doi/10.1136/hrt.66.5.351

[17] COVID-19 Treatment Guidelines Panel. Coronavirus Disease 2019 (COVID-19) Treatment Guidelines. National Institutes of Health. 2019. Available from: https://www.covid19treatmentguidelines.nih.gov/ [Accessed: February 23, 2022]

[18] Wong SH, Lui RN, Sung JJ. Covid-19 and the digestive system. Journal of Gastroenterology and Hepatology. 2020;**35**(5):744-748. Available from: http://www.ncbi.nlm.nih.gov/pubmed/32215956

[19] Lopez Reboiro M, Suarez Fuentetaja R, Gutierrez Lopez R, Ares Castro-Conde B, Sardiña Gonzalez C, Navarro Menendez I, et al. Role of lupus anticoagulant and von Williebrand factor in chronic reactive endothelitis in COVID-19. The Journal of Infection. 2021;**82**:e27-e28

[20] Bowels L, Platton S, Yartey N. Lupus anticoagulant and abnormal coagulation tests in patients with COVID-19. The New England Journal of Medicine. 2020;**383**(3):286-288

[21] Bradbury CA, McQuilten Z. Anticoagulation in COVID-19. Lancet. 2021;**6736**(21):2021-2023

[22] Sociedad Española de Trombosis y Hemostasia. Recomendaciones de tromboprofilaxis y tratamiento antitrombótico en pacientes con COVID-19. Sociedad Española de Trombosis y Hemostasia. 2020:1-8

[23] Zhou F, Yu T, Du R, Fan G, Liu Y, Liu Z, et al. Clinical course and risk factors for mortality of adult inpatients with COVID-19 in Wuhan, China: A retrospective cohort study. Lancet. 2020;**395**(10229):1054-1062. DOI: 10.1016/S0140-6736(20)30566-3

[24] Jorda A, Siller-Matula JM, Zeitlinger M, Jilma B, Gelbenegger G. Anticoagulant treatment regimens in patients with Covid-19: A meta-analysis. Clinical Pharmacology and Therapeutics. 2021;**111**(3):614-623. DOI: 10.1002/cpt.2504

[25] López-Reyes R, Oscullo G, Jiménez D, Cano I, García-Ortega A. Riesgo trombótico y COVID-19: revisión de la evidencia actual para una mejor aproximación diagnóstica y terapéutica. Archivos de Bronconeumología. 2021;**57**: 55-64

[26] National Institutes of Health. Treatment guidelines panel. Coronavirus disease 2019 (COVID-19). NIH. 2021. 2019:1-243. Available from: https://www.covid19treatmentguidelines.nih.gov/

[27] Buijsers B, Yanginlar C, Maciej-Hulme ML, de Mast Q, van der Vlag J. Beneficial non-anticoagulant mechanisms underlying heparin treatment of COVID-19 patients. eBioMedicine. 2020;**59**:102969. Available from: http://www.ncbi.nlm.nih.gov/pubmed/32853989

[28] Ortega-Paz L, Galli M, Capodanno D, Franchi F, Rollini F, Bikdeli B, et al. Safety and efficacy of different prophylactic anticoagulation dosing regimens in critically and non-critically ill patients with COVID-19: A systematic review and meta-analysis of randomized controlled trials. European Heart Journal. Cardiovascular Pharmacotherapy. 2021:1-10. DOI: 10.1093/ehjcvp/pvab070/6370175

[29] Demelo-Rodriguez P, Farfán-Sedano AI, Pedrajas JM, Llamas P, Sigüenza P, Jaras MJ, et al. Bleeding risk in hospitalized patients with COVID-19 receiving intermediate- or therapeutic doses of thromboprophylaxis. Journal of Thrombosis and Haemostasis. 2021;**19**(8):1981-1989

[30] ATTACC Investigators, ACTIV-4a Investigators, REMAP-CAP Investigators, Lawler PR, Goligher EC, Berger JS, et al. Therapeutic anticoagulation with heparin in noncritically ill patients with Covid-19. The New England Journal of Medicine. 2021;**385**(9):790-802. DOI: 10.1056/NEJMoa2105911

[31] Sholzberg M, Tang GH, Rahhal H, Alhamzah M, Kreuziger LB, Áinle FN, et al. Effectiveness of therapeutic heparin versus prophylactic heparin on death, mechanical ventilation, or intensive care unit admission in moderately ill patients with covid-19 admitted to hospital: RAPID randomised clinical trial. BMJ. 2021;**375**:n2400. Available from: http://www.ncbi.nlm.nih.gov/pubmed/34649864

[32] Lopes RD, de Barros E Silva PGM, Furtado RHM, Macedo AVS, Bronhara B, Damiani LP, et al. Therapeutic versus prophylactic anticoagulation for patients admitted to hospital with COVID-19 and elevated D-dimer concentration (ACTION): An open-label, multicentre, randomised, controlled trial. Lancet (London, England). 2021;**397**(10291):2253-2263. Available from: http://www.ncbi.nlm.nih.gov/pubmed/34097856

[33] Marcos-Jubilar M, Carmona-Torre F, Vidal R, Ruiz-Artacho P, Filella D, Carbonell C, et al. Therapeutic versus prophylactic Bemiparin in hospitalized patients with nonsevere COVID-19 pneumonia (BEMICOP study): An open-label, Multicenter, randomized, controlled trial. Thrombosis and Haemostasis. 2022;**122**(02):295-299. Available from: http://www.ncbi.nlm.nih.gov/pubmed/34638151

[34] Spyropoulos AC, Goldin M, Giannis D, Diab W, Wang J, Khanijo S, et al. Efficacy and safety of therapeutic-dose heparin vs standard prophylactic or intermediate-dose heparins for Thromboprophylaxis in high-risk hospitalized patients with COVID-19: The HEP-COVID randomized clinical trial. JAMA Internal Medicine. 2021;**181**(12):1612-1620

[35] Zhang S, Li Y, Liu G, Su B. Intermediate-to-therapeutic versus prophylactic anticoagulation for coagulopathy in hospitalized COVID-19 patients: A systemic review and meta-analysis. Thrombosis Journal. 2021;**19**(1):1-13

[36] INSPIRATION Investigators, Sadeghipour P, Talasaz AH, Rashidi F, Sharif-Kashani B, Beigmohammadi MT, Farrokhpour M, et al. Effect of intermediate-dose vs standard-dose prophylactic anticoagulation on

thrombotic events, extracorporeal membrane oxygenation treatment, or mortality among patients with COVID-19 admitted to the intensive care unit: The INSPIRATION randomized clinic. JAMA. 2021;**325**(16):1620-1630

Chapter 6

Methodological Quality of Clinical Practice Guidelines for Pharmacological Prophylaxis of Venous Thromboembolism in Hospitalized Adult Medical and Surgical Patients and Summary of the Main Categories of Recommendations Included in High-Quality CPGs: A Systematic Review

Ana Paula Callejo de Souza, Franciele Cordeiro Gabriel, Géssica Caroline Henrique Fontes-Mota, Mariana de Siqueira Siva and Eliane Ribeiro

Abstract

Venous thromboembolism (VTE) is a complex multifactorial disease with an average annual incidence of approximately 1 per 1000 in the adult population. Recommendations about pharmacological prophylaxis of VTE in adult hospitalized surgical and medical patients are available in clinical practice guidelines (CPGs) to optimize healthcare delivery and improve patient outcomes. The aim of this study was to examine the methodological quality of CPGs for pharmacological prophylaxis of VTE in adult hospitalized medical and surgical patients and to summarize the main categories to contextualize the recommendations included in high-quality CPGs. Methodology: The study used the ADAPTE to contextualize in categories the main recommendations of the high-quality CPGs assessed by the Appraisal of Guidelines for Research and Evaluation (AGREE II). Results: Fourteen CPGs were screened for assessment of quality methodology by AGREE II instrument. Seven of fourteen CPGs were selected as high-quality (>60%) across domains 3 and 6 to contextualize the recommendations in categories. Conclusion: Seven CPGs evaluated by AGREE had scores above 60% in domains 3 and 6. The scope addressed by the high-quality CPGs included important aspects of pharmacological prophylaxis of VTE in hospitalized patients.

Keywords: venous thromboembolism, practice guidelines, high-quality, adaptation, systematic review

1. Introduction

Venous thromboembolism (VTE) is a complex multifactorial disease influenced by acquired or inherited predispositions to thrombosis, environmental exposures, and the interaction between them, and can manifest as deep vein thrombosis (DVT) or pulmonary thromboembolism (PTE) [1].

The average annual incidence is approximately 1 per 1000 in the adult population, with a higher incidence rate in men than in women. The incidence increases after the age of 45, reaching a rate of 5 or 6 per 1000 inhabitants annually in the elderly over 80 years [1–3].

Approximately 50% of thrombotic events occur during or shortly after hospitalization, with 24% in surgical patients and 22% in medical patients [1]. PTE accounts for 5-10% of hospitalized patient deaths, making VTE the most common cause of preventable deaths in hospitalized patients, and thromboprophylaxis is an important strategy to improve patient safety in hospitals [4].

Clot formation during hospitalization, surgical procedure, or health care is known as hospital-acquired thrombosis and can occur during hospitalization and up to 90 days after discharge [4]. In addition, VTE is associated with recurrence, post-thrombotic syndrome, chronic pulmonary hypertension, and bleeding due to anticoagulation [1, 5, 6]. These complications substantially contribute to patient morbidity and the cost of management [4].

Although national and international consensus is available, studies show that 50% of at-risk patients do not receive adequate prophylaxis [7]. According to these consensuses for the prevention of VTE induced in hospitals, should take into account the risk factors for the occurrence of an event, the benefits of available prophylactic agents, possible complications, and the cost of treatment, information that should be part of a formal hospital strategy supporting the decision of the professionals involved [8, 9].

Clinical Practice Guidelines (CPGs) are tools that contain recommendations on clinical health interventions, with the aim of improving patient care, based on a systematic review of evidence to assess the benefits and harms of different therapeutic alternatives in health care [10, 11].

The Institute of Medicine (IOM) defines CPGs as "statements that included recommendations, intended to optimize patient care, informed by a systematic review of evidence and an assessment of the benefits and harms of alternative care options". CPGs are underpinned by systematic review evidence and are usually formulated by groups of stakeholders with relevant domain expertise [12].

One way to obtain the CPGs is through adaptation. The ADAPTE Collaboration, an international collaboration of researchers, guideline developers, and guideline implementers, has developed a systematic approach tool for adapting guidelines considering the organizational and cultural environment to application in a different context. In this way, it is possible to take advantage of existing guidelines and produce high-quality adaptation [13].

The use of an instrument to assess the quality of guidelines, the Appraisal of guidelines research and Evaluation (AGREE II), is recommended during the guidelines decision and selection tasks that take place within the adaptation process by the ADAPTE methodology. From the selected CPGs, summaries of recommendations are created, allowing the visualization of whether the recommendations from different CPGs are similar or different, verifying which of these have strong evidence and providing the clinical importance of each one of them [14, 15].

Therefore, the aim of this study was to analyze the methodological quality of CPGs for pharmacological VTE prophylaxis in adult hospitalized medical and surgical patients; and to summarize the main categories of the recommendations included in high-quality CPGs.

1.1 Adaptation of clinical practice guidelines

Adaptation of guidelines is a systematic approach to modify guidelines produced in a cultural place and organizational setting to be applicable in another context [16]. The adaptation is an alternative to the development of a new guideline preserving the principle of evidence-based practice [17].

The ADAPTE collaboration is a group of researchers, guideline developers, and guideline implementers who proposed a systematic approach to adapting guidelines that ensure the elaboration of final recommendations and that address specific health issues adapted to the context of use, meeting local needs, priorities, legislation, policy, and resources [16].

The process is divided into 3 main phases, set up, adaptation and finalization, with 24 steps divided into 9 modules [13]. **Figure 1** demonstrates a summary of the processes.

The Set-up phase is described in 6 steps. At this stage, it must be verified whether the adaptation is feasible, tracking the availability of guidelines in specific repertoires to proceed with the adaptation process. A working group must also be defined with the activities to be developed by each member for the selected topic. All members must have their tasks well described and must sign the conflict-of-interest term. At this stage, it must also be defined how the consensus for decision-making among the members will be carried out, which must be described in the final document. All stages of the set-up phase must be described in the adaptation plan [11, 13, 16].

In the adaptation phase, the clinical questions that guide the search for CPGs must be defined. The search must be carried out with the elaboration of the clinical question. For this purpose, an acronym can be used, for example, PIPOH: Population, Intervention, Professional, Outcome and Health care setting, which allows for defining the clinical question by addressing the aspects necessary for the development of a well-defined search strategy, being able to identify relevant guidelines in databases and guideline-specific repositories, websites of guideline development organizations and specialized societies [11, 13, 16]. **Table 1** describes the components of the acronym.

The quality of the selected guidelines can be evaluated by the AGREE II (http://www.agreetrust.org)instrument,through the 23 items that make up the tool, and evaluate the guideline development method. In addition to quality, experts should be aware of the guidelines' update dates and check whether the recommendations have undergone changes that may impact the adaptation of the CPGs [11, 13].

Another factor to be evaluated is the content of the guidelines, through the extraction of recommendations, with their levels of evidence that must compose the matrices and can be grouped by guideline or by similarity [13].

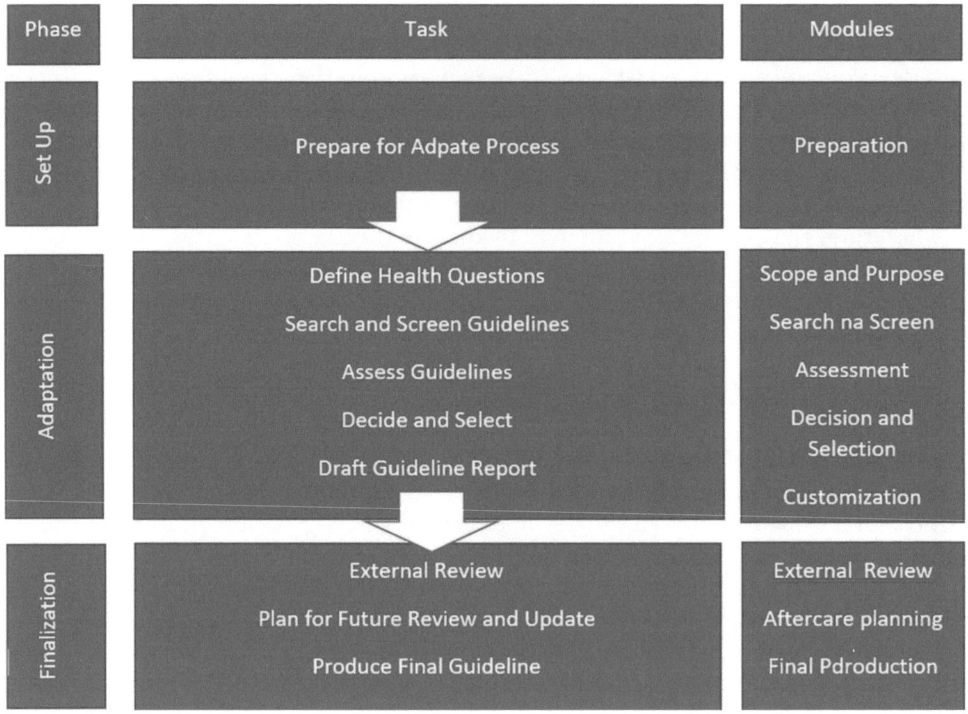

Figure 1.
Summary of the adaptation process from the description of the ADAPTE tool. ADAPTE collaboration (2009) was prepared and adopted by the author [13].

PIPOH	Description
Population	Characteristics of the disease or condition for the population of interest
Intervention	Intervention of interest
Professional	Professionals targeted by the guideline
Outcome	Expected outcomes
Health system	Location where the guideline will be implemented

Table 1.
Description of the PIPOH acronym for the elaboration of the clinical question ADAPTE collaboration (2009) prepared and adapted by the author [13].

The recommendations help the end-user of the CPGs by describing what should be done to make an appropriate decision in certain situations and optimize patient care to improve the health outcome both individually and collectively [13].

The acceptability and applicability of recommendations to the target context depend on the adaptation to variables such as availability and organization of health services, resources, beliefs, and values of the population. All details of the process must be recorded in a draft document [11, 13].

In the finalization phase, the external review process by users must take place. Thus, all comments received must be evaluated by the elaboration group that proceeds with the modification of the guideline, if pertinent. Every process must also be documented. At this stage, the guideline update plan should also be considered. With all the prerequisites defined, the final version can be produced and deployed [13].

1.2 Quality assessment of clinical practice guidelines

Adaptation involves the step of critically evaluating the methodological quality of the CPGs for the selection of high-quality guidelines, determined by confidence in how potential biases in the elaboration process were addressed and by verifying the validity of recommendations for clinical practice considering the risks, benefits, and costs [11, 13].

The first version of the Appraisal of Guidelines Research and Evaluation (AGREE) was published in 2003 by the AGREE collaboration, a group of international guidelines developers and researchers, with the aim of obtaining a tool for assessing the quality of CPGs. The evaluation included a judgment of the methods used to develop the guidelines, the components of the final recommendations, and the factors that are linked to their implementation. The instrument was translated into several languages and quickly became accepted as a gold standard tool for guideline evaluation. It has been tested in 11 countries in more than 100 guidelines and with more than 200 evaluators, being endorsed by the World Health Organization, the Council of Europe, and the Guideline International Network (GIN). The revised version was published in 2009 [15].

All 23 items on the instrument are scored on a Likert scale from one to seven, where one is "strongly disagree" and seven is "strongly agree". Scores between 2 and 6 are assigned when the item does not meet all criteria and considerations [15]. In this way, each domain is scored according to the dimension of quality addressed as described in **Table 2**.

The quality score is calculated for each of the six domains independently, which receives a score ranging from 0 to 100%. The calculation is performed by adding the

Domain	Definition
Scope and purpose	In this domain, the objective of the CPG, the correct elaboration of clinical questions, and the description of the target population of the guideline are evaluated (items 1-3)
Stakeholder involvement	Concerns about the professionals involved in the development process, addressing patient preferences, and defining target users (items 4-6)
Rigor of development	The evidence search strategy, classification of the level of evidence of the selected studies, mechanisms for formulating recommendations, whether there was an external review, and whether there are plans to update the GPC are evaluated (item 7-14)
Clarity of presentation	In this domain, it is evaluated whether the recommendations are clearly described, whether the guide considers different possibilities for managing the disease and whether the key recommendations are easily located (item 15 – 17)
Applicability	It addresses the description of barriers and facilitators that impact the applicability of the guideline and brings suggestions of tools and resources spent to apply the GPC and monitoring indicators (item 18-21)
Editorial independence	Evaluates the description of the financing funds and their impact on the preparation of the guideline and the existence of the conflict-of-interest policy (item 22-23)

Table 2.
Domains of the AGREE II instrument. AGREE next steps consortium (2017), prepared and adapted by the author [15].

scores of the individual items and calculating the maximum and minimum scores that the domain could receive depending on the number of evaluators, with at least two being indicated [15]. The calculation of the score for each domain does not indicate that one domain is more relevant than the other. The AGREE II manual also does not set a limit to distinguish between high- and low-quality CPGs [18, 19].

2. Methodology

The study involves a systematic search for CPGs for pharmacological prophylaxis of VTE in adult hospitalized orthopedic and non-orthopedic surgical patients and pharmacological prophylaxis of VTE in adult hospitalized patients with acutely ill medical. To summarize the main topics in the recommendations of the high-quality CPGs the ADAPTE methodology was used.

2.1 Selection criteria

The first step was formulating the clinical question grounded on the acronym PIPOH as described in **Table 3**.

The clinical question guided the search for CPGs through the definition of descriptors and inclusion criteria. The following items were outside the scope of this study: pregnant and postpartum women, pediatric patients, outpatients, patients being treated for VTE, and patients suspected or diagnosed with COVID-19. The search included CPGs defined by the IOM [12] open access, in updated versions in English, Portuguese and Spanish, published between 2011 and 2021. The study was registered on the protocol registration portal, International Register of Systematic Review (PROSPERO), under number CRD42021232578.

2.2 Bibliographic databases

An electronic database search was conducted in April 2021 by CPGs for pharmacological prophylaxis in adult hospitalized patients published between January 1, 2011, and March 31, 2021. A search strategy was developed using the keywords "venous thromboembolism" and "guideline" in the following databases: Medline (via Pubmed), Cochrane Library (via CENTRAL), Embase, and Lilacs, and on specific CPG repositories and organization websites: Australian Clinical Practice guidelines

PIPOH	Inclusion criteria
Population	Adults (> 18 years) and hospitalized (> 24 hours)
Intervention	Pharmacological prophylaxis for venous thromboembolism (VTE)
Professional	Multi-professional team of a hospital
Outcome	Prophylaxis of VTE in 1) orthopedic and non -orthopedic surgical patients; 2) acutely ill medical patients
Health system	Hospital

Table 3.
Description of the PIPOH acronym for the elaboration of the clinical question for pharmacological prophylaxis of VTE in adult hospitalized patients.

(clinicalguidelines.gov.au), Canadian Agency for Drugs and Technologies in Health (cadth.ca), International Guidelines Network (gin.net), ECRI Guidelines Trust (guide lines.ecri.org), Scottish Intercollegiate Guidelines Network (sign.ac.uk), Queensland Health (health.qld.gov.au), American Society of Hematology (hematology.org), American College of physicians (acponline.org), American College of chest physicians (chestnet.org), International Union of Angiology (angiology.org), National Institute

Databases	Strategy search
Medline (via Pubmed)	("Practice Guidelines as Topic"[MeSH Terms] OR ("Practice Guidelines as Topic"[MeSH Terms] OR ("practice"[All Fields] AND "guidelines"[All Fields] AND "topic"[All Fields]) OR "Practice Guidelines as Topic"[All Fields] OR ("clinical"[All Fields] AND "guidelines"[All Fields] AND "topic"[All Fields])) OR ("Practice Guidelines as Topic"[MeSH Terms] OR ("practice"[All Fields] AND "guidelines"[All Fields] AND "topic"[All Fields]) OR "Practice Guidelines as Topic"[All Fields] OR ("best"[All Fields] AND "practices"[All Fields]) OR "best practices"[All Fields]) OR ("Practice Guidelines as Topic"[MeSH Terms] OR ("practice"[All Fields] AND "guidelines"[All Fields] AND "topic"[All Fields]) OR "Practice Guidelines as Topic"[All Fields] OR ("best"[All Fields] AND "practice"[All Fields]) OR "best practice"[All Fields]) OR ("Practice Guideline"[Publication Type] OR ("Practice Guideline"[Publication Type] OR "Practice Guidelines as Topic"[MeSH Terms] OR "clinical practice guideline"[All Fields]) OR (("ambulatory care facilities"[MeSH Terms] OR ("ambulatory"[All Fields] AND "care"[All Fields] AND "facilities"[All Fields]) OR "ambulatory care facilities"[All Fields] OR "clinic"[All Fields] OR "clinic s"[All Fields] OR "clinical"[All Fields] OR "clinically"[All Fields] OR "clinicals"[All Fields] OR "clinics"[All Fields]) AND ("Guideline"[Publication Type] OR "guidelines as topic"[MeSH Terms] OR "guidelines"[All Fields]))) OR "Guideline"[Publication Type]) AND ("Venous Thromboembolism"[MeSH Terms] OR ("Venous Thromboembolism"[MeSH Terms] OR ("venous"[All Fields] AND "thromboembolism"[All Fields]) OR "Venous Thromboembolism"[All Fields] OR ("thromboembolism"[All Fields] AND "venous"[All Fields]) OR "thromboembolism venous"[All Fields]))
Embase	('practice guideline'/exp./mj OR 'clinical practice guidelines'/mj OR 'guidelines'/mj OR 'guidelines as topic'/mj OR 'practice guideline'/mj OR 'practice guidelines'/mj OR 'practice guidelines as topic'/mj) AND ('venous thromboembolism'/exp. OR 'thromboembolism, venous' OR 'vein thromboembolism' OR 'venous thromboembolism') AND [2011–2021]/py AND [embase]/lim
Cochrane	#1 Mesh descriptor: [Venous Thromboembolism] explode all trees
	#2 (Thromboembolism, Venous)
	#3 #1 OR #2
	#4 MeSH descriptor: [Practice Guidelines as Topic] explode all trees
	#5 Clinical Guidelines as Topic) OR (Best Practices) OR (Best Practice) OR (Practice Guideline) OR (Clinical Guidelines) OR (Guideline)
	#6 #4 OR #5
	#7 #3 AND #6
LILACS	"TROMBOEMBOLISMO" or "TROMBOEMBOLISMO VENOSO" [Palavras] and (("GUIDELINE" or "GUIDELINE/PROTOCOL" or "GUIDELINES AS TOPIC" or "GUIDELINES/CONSENSUS") or "GUIA DE PRATICA CLINICA" or "GUIA DE PRATICA MEDICA") or "DIRETRIZ" or "DIRETRIZ DE PRATICA MEDICA" or "DIRETRIZ PARA A PRATICA CLINICA" or "DIRETRIZ PARA A PRATICA MEDICA" or "DIRETRIZ/PROTOCOLO" [Palavras]

Table 4.
Search strategy used in PubMed, Cochrane library, Embase, and Lilacs databases.

for Health and care Excellence (nice.org.uk), National Guidelines Clearing House (guidelines.gov), European Society of Anesthesiology and intensive care (esaic.org), Thrombosis Canada (thrombosiscanada.ca). Search strategies are described in **Table 4**.

2.3 Selection process

Two reviewers independently screened the retrieve titles and abstracts. After the first screening two reviewers screened the full text independently and a third reviewer resolves disagreements when there was no consensus. All screenings were conducted by importing the search results into the Rayyan ® reference manager.

2.4 Clinical practice guideline quality assessment

Three reviewers trained in the AGREE II instrument, conduct an independently quality assessment of each eligible CPG. The instrument consists of 23 items grouped in six domains. Each item receives three grades one from each reviewer directly on the online platform My AGREE Plus (http://www.agreetrust.org). The grades were considered discrepant when there was a difference of two or more points between the reviewers' grades. Discrepancies in the scoring were resolved by group discussions. For defining a high-quality CPG was used the AGREE II domain scores and a cut-off of 60% or more for 3 (rigor of development) and 6 (editorial independence) AGREE II domains [19].

2.5 Summary of the recommendations in categories included in the clinical practice guidelines

After the quality assessment of each eligible CPGs, those who scored higher than 60% in 3 (rigor of development) and 6 (editorial independence) AGREE II domains were used to summarize the recommendations in categories included in the CPGs.

Two reviewers independently read each CPG to gain an overall knowledge of content and identify topics covered by the guidelines. The topics with the same theme were defined through constant comparison and were grouped within categories to contextualize the recommendations for pharmacological VTE prophylaxis. Generic recommendations were not included within the categories.

3. Results

3.1 Identification of CPGs

The bibliographic search identified 4698 records from databases of which 478 were duplicates. It was screened 4220 remaining references by title and abstract and excluded 4064 that were not in the selection criteria. It was reviewed, 156 documents in full text, and excluded 142 documents. Fourteen CPGs were included. **Figure 2** displays the selection process through the PRISMA statement flow diagram [20].

3.2 Methodological quality of clinical practice guidelines

The AGREE II standardized domain ratings are summarized in **Table 5**.

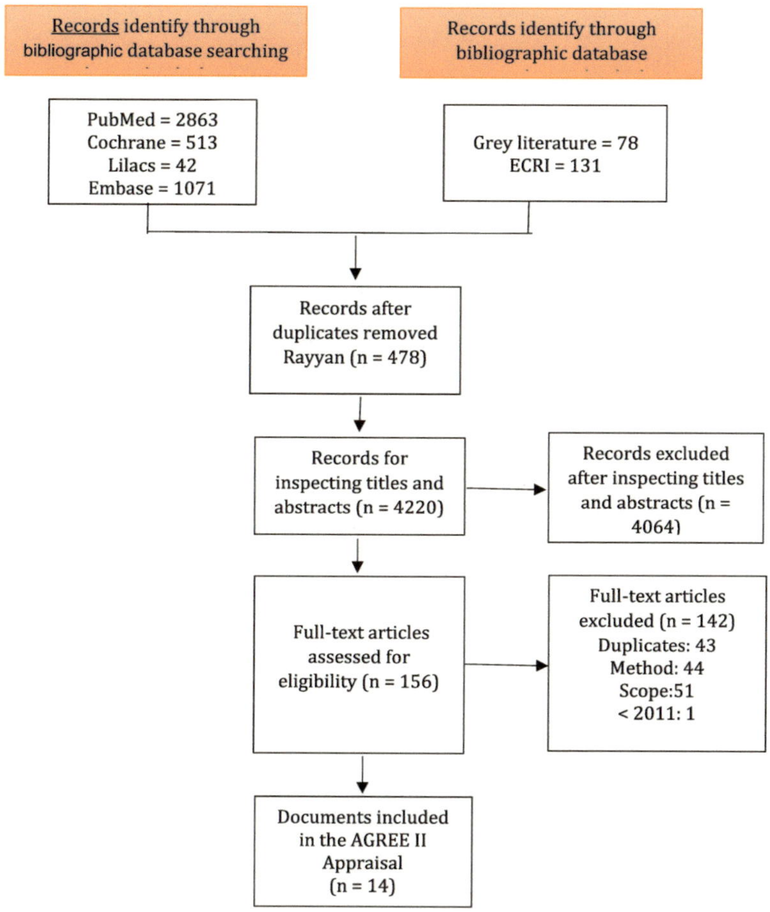

Figure 2.
PRISMA flow diagram of study selection.

01. National Institute for Health and Care Excellence (NICE, 2018): Venous thromboembolism in over 16 s Reducing the risk of hospital-acquired deep vein thrombosis or pulmonary embolism; 02. American Society of Hematology (ASH, 2018): American Society of Hematology guidelines for the management of venous thromboembolism: Prevention of venous thromboembolism in surgical and medical hospitalized patients; 03. Scottish Intercollegiate Guidelines Network (SIGN, 2014): Prevention and management of venous thromboembolism; 04. German interdisciplinary, evidence- and consensus-based (S3, 2015): Clinical practice guideline: The prophylaxis of venous thromboembolism; 05. National Health and Medical Research Council (NHMRC, 2012): Clinical practice guideline for the prevention of venous thromboembolism in patients admitted to Australian hospitals; 06. American College of Chest Physicians (ACCP, 2012): Antithrombotic Therapy and Prevention of Thrombosis, 9th ed.: American College of Chest Physicians Evidence-Based Clinical Practice Guidelines; 07. American College Physicians (ACP, 2011): Venous thromboembolism prophylaxis in hospitalized patients: A clinical practice guideline from the American College of Physicians; 08. Saudi Scientific Hematology Society and the Saudi Association for VTE (SAVTE, 2013): Saudi Arabian Handbook for Healthcare

	Clinical Practice Guidelines	Domain 1	Domain 2	Domain 3	Domain 4	Domain 5	Domain 6
		Scope and Purpose	Stakeholder Involvement	Rigor of Development	Clarity of Presentation	Applicability	Editorial Independence
01	NICE, 2018 [21]	93%	76%	86%	83%	64%	83%
02	ASH, 2018 [22, 23]	80%	74%	76%	81%	58%	86%
03	SIGN, 2014 [24]	81%	80%	72%	81%	61%	69%
04	S3, 2015 [25]	74%	65%	72%	74%	35%	83%
05	NHRMC, 2012 [26]	80%	78%	72%	78%	49%	61%
06	ACCP, 2012 [27–29]	80%	54%	67%	83%	38%	75%
07	ACP, 2011 [8]	76%	56%	65%	63%	28%	67%
08	SAVTE, 2013 [30]	67%	50%	54%	70%	58%	50%
09	IUA, 2013 [31]	59%	30%	47%	59%	33%	33%
10	Queensland Health, 2018 [32]	83%	52%	44%	72%	67%	44%
11	Mexicano, 2011 [33]	57%	31%	40%	65%	17%	8%
12	MOH, 2013 [34]	80%	54%	39%	76%	35%	61%
13	Argentina, 2013 [35]	50%	46%	35%	57%	18%	44%
14	JCS, 2011 [36]	44%	31%	19%	43%	17%	0%

Table 5.
AGREE II standardized domain scores for the 14 included CPGs for pharmacological prophylaxis of VTE in hospitalized adult surgical and medical patients.

Guideline Development; 09. International Union Angiology (IUA, 2013): Prevention and Treatment of Venous Thromboembolism; 10. Medication Services (Queensland Health, 2018): Guideline for the Prevention of Venous Thromboembolism (VTE) in Adult Hospitalized Patients; 11. Colégio Mexicano de Ortopedia y Traumatología (Mexicano, 2011): Declaración de posición conjunta del Colegio Mexicano de Ortopedia y Traumatología: Profilaxis de la enfermedad tromboembólica venosa en cirugía ortopédica de alto riesgo; 12. Ministry of Health of Malaysia (MOH, 2013): Clinical Practice Guidelines: Prevention and Treatment of Venous Thromboembolism; 13. Researchers Group (Argentina, 2013): Guía de recomendaciones para la profilaxis de la enfermedad tromboembólica venosa en adultos en la Argentina; 14. Japanese Circulation Society (JCS, 2011): Guidelines for the Diagnosis, Treatment, and Prevention of Pulmonary Thromboembolism and Deep Vein Thrombosis;

The methodological quality of fourteen (14) CPGs was assessed by AGREE II instrument. Seven (50%) guidelines obtained scores equal to or greater than 60% in domains 3 or 6 being considered of high quality as described in **Table 6**. The mean scores for the domains were: scope and purpose 72%, stakeholder involvement 56%, rigor of development 56%, clarity of presentation 70%, applicability 41%, and editorial Independence 55%.

	Clinical practice guideline	Name	Organization	Country
01	NICE, 2018 [21]	Venous thromboembolism in over 16 s Reducing the risk of hospital-acquired deep vein thrombosis or pulmonary embolism	National Institute for Health and Care Excellence	United Kingdom
02	ASH, 2018 [22, 23]	Guideline for management of venous thromboembolism: Prevention of venous thromboembolism in surgical and medical hospitalized patients	American Society of Hematology	United States
03	SIGN, 2014 [24]	Prevention and management of venous thromboembolism	Scottish Intercollegiate Guidelines Network	Scotland
04	S3, 2015 [25]	Clinical practice guideline: The prophylaxis of venous thromboembolism	German interdisciplinary, evidence- and consensus-based	German
05	NHRMC, 2012 [26]	Clinical practice guidelines for the prevention of venous thromboembolism in patients admitted to Australian hospitals	National Health and Medical Research Council	Australia
06	ACCP, 2012 [27–29]	Antithrombotic Therapy and Prevention of Thrombosis, 9th ed.: American College of Chest Physicians Evidence-Based Clinical Practice Guidelines	American College of Chest Physicians	United States
07	ACP, 2011 [8]	Venous thromboembolism prophylaxis in hospitalized patients: A clinical practice guideline from the American College of Physicians	American College Physicians	United States

Table 6.
Clinical practice guidelines for pharmacological prophylaxis of VTE in hospitalized adult medical and surgical patients with high quality assessed by AGREE II.

3.3 Summary of the recommendations in categories

Six major categories, included in high-quality CPGs, were considered important to contextualize the recommendations. There were: 1. patient involvement, 2. risk of VTE and bleeding, 3. indication and strategy of pharmacological prophylaxis in acute ill medical patients, 4. indication and strategy of pharmacological prophylaxis in orthopedic surgical patients, 5. indication and strategy of pharmacological prophylaxis in no-orthopedic surgical patients, 6. monitoring adverse effects.

3.3.1 Patient involvement

- Giving Information: Three [21, 24, 25] of the seven (43%) guidelines included recommendations for giving information to the patients about the importance of VTE prophylaxis on admission.

- Planning Discharge: Three [21, 24, 25] of the seven (43%) included recommendations for planning discharge.

3.3.2 Risk of VTE and bleeding

- Risk Assessment of VTE and bleeding: Five [8, 21, 24–26] of the seven (71%) guidelines included recommendations for identifying the risk of VTE and bleeding in medical and surgical patients admitted to the hospital.

- Reassessment of risk of VTE and bleeding: Two [21, 24] of the seven (29%) guidelines included recommendations about reassessment periodically of the risk of VTE and bleeding in medical and surgical patients admitted to the hospital.

- Risk Assessment Tools: Four [21, 24–26] of the seven (57%) guidelines included recommendations about risk assessment tools. The CPGs discuss assessment tools for VTE and bleeding to perform the risk factors. The factors are related to exposure (type of surgical procedure/trauma/acute disease, extent of immobilization) and disposition (individual inherited and acquired factors) [25] and to estimate the baseline risk for patients with low and high VTE risk, has been used data from risk assessment models (RAMs) [27–29]. These tools have limitations including lack of prospective validation, applicability only to high-risk subgroups, inadequate follow-up time, and excessive complexity [27–29].

3.3.3 Indication and strategy of pharmacological prophylaxis in acute ill medical patients

- Pharmacological prophylaxis: Six [8, 21, 24–26, 29] of the seven (86%) included guidelines with recommendations to pharmacological thromboprophylaxis. CPGs report that after individually assessing for risk of VTE and bleeding and the assessment favors the use of pharmacologic thromboprophylaxis, the use of pharmacological agents has been considered.

- Pharmacological agents: All guidelines [8, 21, 23–26, 29] contained recommendations related pharmacological agents for patients who receive pharmacological prophylaxis. Of these seven guidelines, three [21, 24, 25] contained recommendations for pharmacological VTE prophylaxis for people with renal impairment or obesity.

- Duration of prophylaxis: Four [21, 24, 25, 29] of the seven (57%) contained recommendations related to the duration of prophylaxis in acute ill medical patients.

4. Indication and strategy of pharmacological prophylaxis in orthopedic surgical patients

ACCP, 2012 [27] classified hip arthroplasty, knee arthroplasty, and hip fracture surgery as major orthopedic surgery. ASH, 2019 [22] recommendations 1 to 8 for patients undergoing major surgery were not included (generic recommendations). ACP, 2011 [8] contained recommendations only for medical patients.

4.1 Hip Arthroplasty

- Pharmacological agents and duration of prophylaxis: Six [21, 22, 24–27] of the seven (86%) guidelines contained recommendations related to pharmacological prophylaxis strategy for surgical patients undergoing hip arthroplasty with high VTE risk determined after individually assess for risk of VTE and bleeding.

- Preoperatively and postoperatively: Only ACCP, 2012 [27] and S3, 2015 [25] contained recommendations for patients undergoing hip arthroplasty preoperatively and postoperatively.

4.2 Knee arthroplasty

- Pharmacological agents and duration of prophylaxis: Six [21, 22, 24–27] of the seven (86%) guidelines contained recommendations related to pharmacological prophylaxis for surgical patients undergoing knee arthroplasty whose risk of VTE outweighs the risk of bleeding determined after to individually assess for risk of VTE and bleeding.

- Preoperatively and postoperatively: Only ACCP, 2012 [27] and S3, 2015 [25] contained recommendations for patients undergoing knee arthroplasty preoperatively and postoperatively.

4.3 Fragility fractures of the pelvis, hip, and proximal femur

- Pharmacological agents and duration of prophylaxis: Five [21, 22, 25–27] of seven (71%) CPGs contained recommendations for patients undergoing surgery for fragility fractures in the absence of contraindications.

- Preoperatively and postoperatively: Only Nice, 2018 [21] and S3, 2015 [25] contained recommendations related to preoperatively and postoperatively in patients undergoing surgery for fragility fractures.

4.4 Foot and ankle orthopedic surgery

Only one guideline [21] considered recommendations for pharmacological prophylaxis in patients undergoing foot or ankle surgery after individually assessing for risk of VTE and bleeding.

4.5 Upper limb orthopedic surgery

Two [21, 25] of seven (29%) CPGs contained recommendations with pharmacological prophylaxis in patients undergoing surgery upper limb surgery.

4.6 Lower limb immobilization

Five [21, 24–27] of seven (71%) CPGs contained recommendations for patients with lower limb immobilization whose risk of VTE outweighs the risk of bleeding and are subject to prolonged immobility.

4.7 Knee arthroscopy

Four [21, 25–27] of seven (57%) CPGs contained recommendations for pharmacological prophylaxis in patients undergoing knee arthroscopy in longer arthroscopic procedures with no contraindications.

5. Indication and strategy of pharmacological prophylaxis no orthopedic surgical patients

5.1 Trauma patients

Five [21, 22, 25–27] of seven (71%) CPGs included recommendations about pharmacological prophylaxis in major trauma patients after assessment to identify the risk of VTE and bleeding.

5.2 General and abdominal-pelvic surgery

This group included patients undergoing gastrointestinal, urological, and gynecologic surgeries. Six [21, 22, 24–26, 28] of the seven (86%) CPGs included recommendations about pharmacological prophylaxis in patients undergoing general and pelvic abdominal surgery depending on the type of risk (low, moderate, or high) after an individual assessment.

5.3 Thoracic surgery

Five [21, 24–26, 28] of the seven (71%) CPGs included recommendations for thoracic surgery after an individual risk assessment. Not included recommendations in cardiac surgery.

5.4 Vascular surgery

This group included recommendations for patients undergoing a lower limb amputation and varicose vein surgery. Six [21, 22, 24–26, 28] of the seven (86%) CPGs included recommendations for pharmacological prophylaxis in patients whose risk of VTE outweighs the risk of bleeding.

5.5 Laparoscopic surgery

Laparoscopic surgery can include procedures ranging from a very short diagnostic laparoscopic procedure to lengthy major surgery, e.g., laparoscopic colectomy. Three [22, 24, 25] CPGs of the seven (43%) included recommendations about pharmacological prophylaxis for patients with risk factors for VTE.

6. Monitoring adverse effects

Heparin-induced thrombocytopenia (HIT) is a serious complication of heparin anticoagulant therapy and can cause thrombocytopenia, venous or arterial thrombosis, skin lesions, and rarely a systemic reaction that can be serious and fatal. HIT may occur in any patient who is receiving heparin [24]. Three [24–26] CPGs of the seven (43%) included recommendation to minimize the incidence of HIT, monitor the development of HIT, and therapeutic options for thrombotic event related to HIT. The ACCP, 2012 [37] and ASH, 2018 [38] have supplementary material that included recommendations about HIT and were not included in this study.

7. Conclusion

This systematic review analyzed the methodological quality and summarized the main recommendations of the CPGs for pharmacological prophylaxis of VTE in adult hospitalized surgical and medical patients.

Seven CPGs were considered with high-quality after assessment by AGREE II a tool accepted as a gold standard for guideline evaluation. The scores with a cut-off of 60% or more for domains 3 (rigor of development) and 6 (editorial independence) were used to identify high-quality CPGs in this study. Domain 3 indicates minimum bias and evidence-based guideline development and domain 6 indicates the relevance of conflict of guideline authors as a potential source of bias. Special attention should be directed to domain 5 (applicability) which indicates the description of barriers and facilitators that impact the applicability of the guideline and had an average score of a 41%. The findings, by presenting the weaknesses in the method's rigor, can also help developers to improve the quality of future CPGs.

Regarding the scope addressed by the guidelines, it was identified that the topics were included regarding important aspects in pharmacological prophylaxis of VTE in hospitalized patients. Most CPGs included recommendations about drug, dose, and duration of therapy that were summarized in the indication and strategy of pharmacological prophylaxis.

The high-quality CPGs discussed about the patient assessment to determine risk stratification for VTE and most CPGs agree that tools have limitations and an individual risk assessment was necessary to focus on patient-specific characteristics, incorporating surgery-specific risk in addition to medical factors. These recommendations were summarized into the risk of VTE and bleeding risk categories.

Some high-quality CPGs included recommendations about the involvement of the patient and family in the management of the prophylaxis of VTE and monitoring adverse effects during the use of the pharmacological prophylaxis. These recommendations were summarized in the category of patient involvement and monitoring adverse effects respectively.

Thus, analyzing the methodological quality and summarizing the recommendations were important steps to support the process of adopting new guidelines for pharmacological prophylaxis of VTE in adult hospitalized surgical and medical patients.

Conflict of interest

Authors have a link only with the University of São Paulo.

Author details

Ana Paula Callejo de Souza*, Franciele Cordeiro Gabriel,
Géssica Caroline Henrique Fontes-Mota, Mariana de Siqueira Siva and Eliane Ribeiro
Departamento de Farmácia, da Faculdade de Farmácia, Universidade de São Paulo,
São Paulo, Brasil

*Address all correspondence to: anapcs@hu.usp.br

References

[1] Darzi AJ et al. Risk-assessment models for VTE and bleeding in hospitalized medical patients: An overview of systematic reviews. Blood Advances. 2020;**4**(19):4929-4944. DOI: 10.1182/BLOODADVANCES.2020002482

[2] Phillippe HM. Overview of venous thromboembolism. The American Journal of Managed Care. 2017;**23**(20): S376-S382. DOI: 10.4103/0019-5049.144643.FIGURE

[3] Heit JA, Spencer FA, White RH. The epidemiology of venous thromboembolism. Journal of Thrombosis and Thrombolysis. 2016; **41**(1):3-14. DOI: 10.1007/s11239-015-1311-6

[4] Cohen AT et al. Venous thromboembolism risk and prophylaxis in the acute hospital care setting (ENDORSE study): A multinational cross-sectional study. Lancet. 2008;**371**: 387-394

[5] Hunt BJ. The prevention of hospital-acquired venous thromboembolism in the United Kingdom. British Journal of Haematology. 2009;**144**(5):642-652. DOI: 10.1111/j.1365-2141.2008.07517.x

[6] Anderson FA, Spencer FA. "Risk factors for venous thromboembolism," Circulation. 2003;**107**(SUPPL. 23):1-16. DOI: 10.1161/01.CIR.0000078469.07362.E6

[7] Curtarelli A et al. Profilaxia de tromboembolismo venoso, podemos fazer melhor? Perfil de risco e profilaxia de tromboembolismo venoso em Hospital Universitário do interior do Estado de São Paulo. Journal of Vascular Brasileiro. 2019;**18**:1-9. DOI: 10.1590/1677-5449.004018

[8] Qaseem A, Chou R, Humphrey LL, Starkey M, Shekelle P. Venous thromboembolism prophylaxis in hospitalized patients: A clinical practice guideline from the American College of Physicians. Annals of Internal Medicine. 2011;**155**(9):625-632. DOI: 10.7326/0003-4819-155-9-201111010-00011

[9] Schünemann HJ, Fretheim A, Oxman AD. Improving the use of research evidence in guideline development: 13. Applicability, transferability and adaptation. Health Research Policy and Systems. 2006;**4**:13. DOI: 10.1186/1478-4505-4-25

[10] Fervers B, Carretier J, Bataillard A. Clinical practice guidelines. Journal of Visceral Surgery. 2010;**147**(6):e341-e349. DOI: 10.1016/j.jviscsurg.2010.10.010

[11] Fervers B et al. Adaptation of clinical guidelines: Literature review and proposition for a framework and procedure. International Journal for Quality in Health Care. 2006;**18**(3):167-176. DOI: 10.1093/intqhc/mzi108

[12] Daley B, Hitman G, Fenton N, Mclachlan S. Assessment of the methodological quality of local clinical practice guidelines on the identification and management of gestational diabetes. BMJ Open. 2019;**9**(6):1-9. DOI: 10.1136/bmjopen-2018-027285

[13] The ADAPTE Collaboration. The ADAPTE Process: Resource Toolkit for Guideline Adaptation. Version 2.0. 2009. pp. 2-95. Available from: http://www.g-i-n.net

[14] Dos Reis EC, Passos SRL, Dos Santos MAB. Quality assessment of clinical guidelines for the treatment of obesity in

adults: Application of the AGREE II instrument. Cad. Saude Publica. 2018;**34**(6). DOI: 10.1590/0102-311X00050517

[15] Brouwers M, Kho ME, Browman GP, Cluzeau F, Feder G, Fervers B, et al. AGREE II: Advancing guideline development, reporting and evaluation in health care. CMAJ. 2010;**182**(18): E839-E842

[16] Attia A. Adaptation of international evidence based clinical practice guidelines: The ADAPTE process. Middle East Fertility Society Journal. 2013;**18**(2): 123-126. DOI: 10.1016/j.mefs.2013.03.002

[17] Donaldson R, Ricciardi L, Sheridan W, Tartaglia S. Textbook of Patient Safety and Clinical Risk Management. Germany: Springer; 2021

[18] World Health Organization. WHO handbook for guideline development. Geneva, Switzerland: World Health Organization; 2014

[19] Hoffmann-Eßer W, Siering U, Neugebauer EAM, Lampert U, Eikermann M. Systematic review of current guideline appraisals performed with the Appraisal of Guidelines for Research & Evaluation II instrument—a third of AGREE II users apply a cut-off for guideline quality. Journal of Clinical Epidemiology. 2018;**95**:120-127. DOI: 10.1016/j.jclinepi.2017.12.009

[20] Page MJ et al. The PRISMA 2020 statement: An updated guideline for reporting systematic reviews. BMJ. 2021;**372**. DOI: 10.1136/bmj.n71

[21] National Institute for Health and Care Excellence (NICE). Venous Thromboembolism in Over 16s: Reducing the Risk of Hospital-Acquired Deep Vein Thrombosis or Pulmonary Embolism. Vol. 2. London: NICE; 2018. pp. 15-32

[22] Anderson DR et al. American Society of Hematology 2019 guidelines for management of venous thromboembolism: Prevention of venous thromboembolism in surgical and medical hospitalized patients. Blood Advances. 2019;**3**(23):3898-3944. DOI: 10.1182/bloodadvances.2019000975

[23] Schünemann HJ et al. American Society of Hematology 2018 guidelines for management of venous thromboembolism: Prophylaxis for hospitalized and non-hospitalized medical patients. Blood Advances. 2018;**2**(22):3198-3225. DOI: 10.1182/bloodadvances.2018022954

[24] Kessler CM. Prevention and management of venous thromboembolism. Clinical Advances in Hematology and Oncology. 2011;**9**(1):9-11 Available from: www.sign.ac.uk

[25] Encke A, Haas S, Kopp I. Clinical practice guideline: The prophylaxis of venous thromboembolism. Deutsches Ärzteblatt International. 2016;**113**(31–32):532-538. DOI: 10.3238/arztebl.2016.0532

[26] National Health and Medical Research Council (Australia), Clinical practice guideline for the prevention of venous thromboembolism in patients admitted to Australian hospitals. United States: National Health and Medical Research Council; 2009

[27] Falck-Ytter Y et al. Prevention of VTE in orthopedic surgery patients. Antithrombotic therapy and prevention of thrombosis, 9th ed: American College of Chest Physicians evidence-based clinical practice guidelines. Chest. 2012;**141**(2 SUPPL):e278S-e325S. DOI: 10.1378/chest.11-2404

[28] Gould MK et al. Prevention of VTE in no orthopedic surgical patients. Antithrombotic therapy and prevention of thrombosis, 9th ed: American College of Chest Physicians evidence-based clinical practice guidelines. Chest. 2012; **141**(2 SUPPL):e227S-e277S. DOI: 10.1378/chest.11-2297

[29] Kahn SR et al. Prevention of VTE in nonsurgical patients. Antithrombotic therapy and prevention of thrombosis, 9th ed: American College of Chest Physicians evidence-based clinical practice guidelines. Chest. 2012;**141**(2 SUPPL):e195S-e226S. DOI: 10.1378/chest.11-2296

[30] Schunemann H, Mustafa R, Brozek J, Carrasco-Labra A, Brignardello-Peterson R. Saudi Arabian Handbook for Healthcare Guideline Development. United States: The Saudi Center for Evidence Based Health Care; 2014

[31] Cardiovascular Disease Educational and Research Trust; European Venous Forum; North American Thrombosis Forum; International Union of Angiology; Union Internationale du Phlebologie. Prevention and Treatment of Venous Thromboembolism: International Consensus Statement. Clinical and Applied Thrombosis Hemostasis. 2013;**19**(2):116-118. DOI: 10.1177/1076029612474840

[32] Medication Services Queensland, Department of Health. Guideline for the Prevention of Venous Thromboembolism (VTE) in Adult Hospitalised Patients. Australia: Medication Services Queensland, Department of Health; 2018

[33] Meza-Reyes GE et al. Declaración de posición conjunta del Colegio Mexicano de Ortopedia y Traumatología: profilaxis de la enfermedad tromboembólica venosa en cirugía ortopédica de alto riesgo. Acta ortopédica Mex. 2011;**25**(4): 216-222

[34] Ministry of Health Malaysia. Clinical Practice Guidelines: Prevention and Treatment of Venous Thromboembolism. Journal of Thrombosis and Haemostasis. 2013;**11** (1):56-70

[35] Vázquez FJ et al. Guía de recomendaciones para la profilaxis de la enfermedad tromboembólica venosa en adultos en la Argentina. Med. (Buenos Aires). 2013;**73**:1-26

[36] JCS Joint Working Group. "Guidelines for the diagnosis, treatment and prevention of pulmonary thromboembolism and deep vein thrombosis (JCS 2009)". Circulation Journal. Apr 2011;**75**(5):1258-1281. DOI: 10.1253/circj.CJ-88-0010

[37] Linkins LA et al. Treatment and prevention of heparin-induced thrombocytopenia: Antithrombotic therapy and prevention of thrombosis, 9th ed: American College of Chest Physicians evidence-based clinical practice guidelines. Chest. 2012; **141**(2 SUPPL):e495S-e530S. DOI: 10.1378/chest.11-2303

[38] Cuker A et al. American Society of Hematology 2018 guidelines for management of venous thromboembolism: Heparin-induced thrombocytopenia. Blood Advances. 2018;**2**(22):3360-3392. DOI: 10.1182/bloodadvances.2018024489